Liquid Gold

Liquid Gold

A true story about cough syrup addiction
and the horrific consequences that resulted

Vonda Reckner Childress

Edited by John A. Childress

Library of Congress Control Number: 2010905999
ISBN: Softcover   978-1-4500-8647-9

This book was printed in the United States of America.

To order additional copies of this book, contact:
Xlibris Corporation
1-888-795-4274
www.Xlibris.com
Orders@Xlibris.com
73757

INTRODUCTION

This book is written from the heart, and details the years—24 of them—that I spent in nearly hopeless drug addiction during what should have been the best years of my life.

I have changed the names of people in this story, including myself. Why? I feel better having the characters speak back to me, and I'd rather not be talking to myself! Obvious reasons for adding fictional names to others are to protect those in my story, so most of the names of people and places are not real. However, the story is mine to the letter, and very little has been altered in the years my book entails.

My memories are vivid; I just hope the facts herein will somehow protect readers who are curious about medicinal drug dependency, because the cost of euphoria is a dear one, including anything life is supposed to mean in a positive sense. Still, if I can overcome this horrific problem (because of God, the right resources and dear, caring people), almost anyone can battle and win the drug war against them. It isn't easy. In fact, it's probably the most difficult climb facing the "hooked". It can be done, and has been conquered by millions of former drug addicts. This is the story of just one, and if it helps just one other person, then I will consider this a success story.

CHAPTER ONE

Kymlin Corell left her censor editing job at the Akron Star & Journal early that spring day in 1985. She couldn't stand the croupy, persistent cough that had bothered her co-workers and kept her from breathing without clearing her throat. She asked to see her doctor, who had an opening that afternoon. Bless him! Dr. Simon York was a family friend, and Kymlin thought she was fortunate in that it probably played a role in the early appointment.

She arrived about 2 p.m., eyes watering and coughing even more frequently. Dr. York had a bedside manner uncommon in the '80s, and, after gently examining her, discovered she was close to pneumonia with a nasty, violent bronchitis. He prescribed a strong cough syrup called Tussionex, which was to be taken once every 12 hours. Upon getting the prescription filled, along with an antibiotic, Kymlin went home to bed. She took a teaspoon of the syrup and lay down, resting until around 9:00 p.m. As evening wore on, her cough became worse, though the cough syrup had helped while she slept. However, it was nearly 2:00 a.m. before she took another teaspoon, since there was supposed to be a 12-hour interval between doses.

"What the heck, I'll take two spoons because I was still coughing after the first one earlier," she thought. "I need to have a good night's sleep because tomorrow is a really big day." All the real estate ads came into the newspaper on Tuesday, and she couldn't afford to miss processing them for the advertising department. She took the second spoonful and lay back down.

She fell asleep for about half an hour, and then awoke with a start. She couldn't understand why she felt so buoyant, so optimistic, so . . . euphoric.

"Wow!" she thought. "I'm really in a good mood, and the bronchitis seems better. I'm going right into the living room to do the TV Guide crossword!"

For this single, free, diligent and smart 33-year-old woman, that crossword was so much fun! She didn't understand the feeling, but she knew darn well she liked it and wouldn't mind its return after it wore off later. She wondered if there was something in the Tussionex or antibiotic that could have so pleasantly rattled her. The "feeling" finally wore off in about three hours. Happy and somehow fulfilled, she returned to bed, yearning for the sudden joyful mood and everything-will-be-all-right sensation. If it was the cough syrup, she would take two more teaspoons tomorrow night and hope for the "feeling," but not in the morning. She didn't know how her work would be affected.

Tuesday was one of the busiest advertising days in recent memory, but Kym didn't notice the overload. She diligently kept doing her work, daydreaming about finding the reason for the "feeling" she would anticipate tonight.

When the long day finally ended, Kym grinned and mumbled something about "earning" the evening to herself and drove home. Even before dinner, she gulped down two teaspoons of the Tussionex, and then hurriedly ate a TV dinner. She had laundry to do, but with the sudden optimism and even anticipation she felt thirty minutes later, she could hardly wait to start the washing machine. Fun! Doing laundry was really enjoyable tonight.

Why hadn't she been given this cough syrup before? It was suppressing her hacking, and giving her a will to live such as she never had before! She understood that she couldn't take it when she would be working, because her co-workers might find her a little ditzy, and she WAS blonde! Ha, ha!

Oh joy, oh rapture! How could a medicine make life so bearable and happy? She didn't know, she didn't care, she was just following doctor's orders, so she was legitimately relishing these past two days. Perhaps she was getting better, she reasoned, but then she knew this feeling had never happened with any other medicine. She would continue to take two teaspoons at night or even when coming home from work, and she would be very happy for several days, because the bottle was eight ounces. Forty-eight teaspoons. She had done the math.

CHAPTER TWO

Life is so amazing, because we plan it out with such precision and then—bingo! The least little footpath takes us into rough waters. Maybe if we realize when that footpath begins, when it starts to cause trouble, we could avoid all the consequences of moving down that footpath. But life has many twists and turns, leading us into bliss, happiness, sorrow and crisis. You never know when that road will offer the good and the bad, and when we should avoid that footpath entirely. Since we don't know the future, we are destined to take the footpath to find out what unexpectedly lay in store.

One thing Kimlyn truly overlooked and virtually ignored during her years of turmoil and tumult which were forthcoming was her spirituality: her relationship with Jesus Christ.

If she had kept the Lord as her Number One priority, the following story may not have occurred. However, when she told that first little white lie about the Tussionex, she opened herself to Satanic influence; she became a tool of the wrong side. She made the cough syrup her first priority and placed God on the back burner for 24 years.

Kimlyn was a Christian believer since the age of 12, when she accepted Jesus as her personal Savior. She had never tried smoking a pot, or any of the recreational and street drugs; to this day she has never smoked a cigarette. She remained close to her family well into her 30s, but all it took to get started down the road to ruin was a seemingly-innocent bottle of cough syrup. It didn't have to be cocaine, meth, angel dust, or heroin to send her life roiling. She didn't have to shoot up or snort anything to change her life drastically. All it took was a teaspoon. A teaspoon excited her beyond words.

Twenty-three days later, she began to be a little concerned. The evenings had been so fun by her or spent with her fiancé Ryan. They had taken in movies, dinner, and conversation a few times during that better part of a month, and Ryan seemed especially cheerful, endearing, and funny. Kym was the happiest she'd ever been, even as a child, and now the medicine was dangerously low. The last evening with Ryan wasn't so blissful, because Kym Corell was worried sick. Her bronchitis was long gone, but her stomach was turning in knots and awful butterflies as she anticipated the end of existence . . . .

"Oh, c'mon, Kym, she told herself. You're still alive! Stop acting like a child whose candy has been denied."

Then she suddenly felt a ray of hope, because the doctor COULD prescribe refills if she were still coughing. Could a little white lie matter when she wanted to continue her life-of-the-party personality?

Dr. York's office opened at 8:30 Wednesday morning, but was only open for a half day. Kym felt a sense of urgency to call at 8:25, but counted the minutes until 8:30. The first three times she heard the answering machine, which was not satisfying her, so she bit her lip and called at 8:40. The wait was horribly tedious.

"Hi, Marlene. This is Kym Corell."

"Oh, yes, Kym. How is your bronchitis?"

"I uh, wish I could say it's never been better, but I can't. I'm still coughing like I've been exposed to a skunk."

"Well, if the cough syrup didn't work, we can prescribe something else . . . . "

"Oh, no—it DID work; it's just that I'm almost out of it. I think it really did help the severity of my cough. Could you prescribe another bottle? I'm sure this will knock it out."

"Um, just a minute, Kym."

What was the problem? Couldn't she just say yes? Oh, perhaps she has to check with Dr. York. Of course she does. I . . . .

"Kym, Dr. York will prescribe one more bottle. He wants you to take it sparingly, okay?"

"Oh, yeah. I know it's got to be strong to fight bronchitis and a cough like mine. Thanks a million, Marlene. And please thank Dr. York for me. I really mean that."

There was a silence, and then Marlene bade Kym goodbye.

Kim was off to the races once again, and she had just as much fun as before. Of course, it was all legitimate, she told herself, except for that little lie about still coughing. But a medicine is a medicine, and, darn it, she wasn't really doing anything wrong. She wasn't trying to get street drugs or anything else she had disdained all her life, like pot, cocaine, and the like. Kym had simply found something that gave her a lift, a mild mood enhancer that made life a little more golden. Golden . . . just like the color of the Tussionex. She had never seen a gold cough syrup before.

For the next three years, bronchitis was an affliction of Kym's, and she was prescribed Tussionex whenever it flared up. If she didn't have it, however, she just dismissed the thought until her next bout with the illness. Then started the really bad near-pneumonia that almost put her in the hospital. She was given three bottles of Tussionex by Dr. York consecutively, and when she asked for the fourth, she was rejected.

"Kymlin, you are taking too much of the cough syrup. I'm beginning to think you are becoming addicted, and there is something like codeine in it," replied Dr. York to her queries.

She knew her days of getting Tussionex from Dr. York were over, and strangely enough, that thought bothered her much more than the idea of addiction did. From that time until now, she thought she could handle the cough syrup and simply quit when her bronchitis was over, but now that she was told point blank that Dr. York would no longer supply her, she became panicky, pulling on her ponytail as the last of her queries was shot down.

Kym was always been known as a bright girl stubbornly holding on to what she wanted, tenaciously refusing to give it up. Even as a baby, she cried for a second bottle of milk in the hospital, her mom had always told others. Now that tenacity would pay off.

She reached for the telephone book and perused the general practice and internal medicine sections, as well as family practice.

Dr. York wasn't the only doctor in town. Her mom had fixed up her first appointment with him several years ago because he had just been divorced, and Mrs. Corell thought perhaps a date with Dr. York might result, but nothing ever did.

Still, Kym liked him as a friend and family practitioner. That was where it stood, and that was fine with her. Ryan was her beau, and he was a darn nice guy with a vice presidential position in the metal stampings plant where he worked. But, back to the phone book . . . .

Oh, yes. Here was Dr. Owen Pirsky, whom her co-worker in advertising visited frequently. Kym had always borne Candice's tales about the drugs she got from Dr. Pirsky for pain, and perhaps cough syrup wouldn't be so difficult to obtain either. She called, made an appointment for her new "cough", and was happy to note it would be tomorrow during her half-day off.

She wrapped up some legal notices and automotive ads, then eagerly raced for her Buick Skylark in the parking deck. There was plenty of time to spare, but this doctor was at least thirty minutes further than the neighboring Dr. York. She arrived there early, filled out papers, then was called in to see Dr. Pirsky by the nurse.

"Hello, young lady, I'm Dr. Pirsky. What seems to be the trouble this afternoon?"

"I have a really terrible cough that is keeping me awake at night, and I think there's been a fever too. I gag a lot with my sensitive gagging reflex, and have almost thrown up."

With her most forlorn look she could muster in her green eyes, she gazed at him.

"Well, we can try an antibiotic; I want to take a look at you first. Then perhaps a good strong cough syrup."

He examined Kim from her eyes to her chest, looking a little puzzled, as he was probably wondering why she felt so bad when he couldn't find anything wrong. Still, she wouldn't have come to him unless she had a legitimate complaint. After all, she was 33 years old, for heaven's sake!

"Fortunately I don't see any pneumonia, but I can prescribe that antibiotic. We'll start with amoxicillin and then some Tessalon perles, and by . . . ."

He was cut off by Kym.

"Oh, uh, those perle things have come open in my throat and I thought I would die! Is a liquid cough syrup possible?"

"I'm puzzled, Kym. I've never heard of that problem before, and the perles seem to have a good reputation. But if you would feel better with a liquid, yes—I'll give you one. Is there anything you are familiar with that has worked in the past?"

"Yes, yes, um . . . I believe so. It's called Tussex or something like that, I think. Sheepishly, she asked, Would that be all right?"

Dr. Pirsky looked into a tiny computer for a moment, then scowled.

"Are you sure it was Tussionex? That's quite strong, all right. It's mostly for very severe pneumonia-type infections and for hard-to-breathe cough spasms only."

She panicked, but insisted that's what she had been given. Perhaps she shouldn't have mispronounced the syrup; the doctor might give her an ineffective one for her needs.

"Please, Doctor, I'm sure it was that Tuss-ion-ex stuff. It REALLY helped. Can I—may I have a little of it?"

"I . . . all right, but just a couple of ounces. You only need to take one teaspoon every 12 hours. Is that how it was before when prescribed?"

"Yes, it was. I hope I haven't been any trouble, but those perles . . . . " She was cut off.

"Don't worry, but please take it sparingly or you could overdo it. This, frankly, is very addictive medicine, and I'm surprised your former doctor prescribed it. You must promise not to ask for a refill, and take it only as needed," he emphasized.

She told him she absolutely would be very careful, etc., etc., etc., when all the time she was thinking about that solitaire, fun evening after work she could have just thirty minutes after taking two teaspoons of the syrup. She said to herself that life is good, fun, and she felt about 20 instead of early 30s.

CHAPTER THREE

"Two teaspoons left, just enough for tonight," she thought as she examined the bottle. A little gold stuff, then what?"

She couldn't go back to Dr. Pirsky because he was about as conservative as they come, and he might suspect something that she did not even suspect about herself yet.

She decided to buy a medicine book to see just why Tussionex was so magical for her. There it was: Tussionex. Okay, what was the potion all about? She read, "hydrocodone and chlorpheniramine (narcotic and antihistamine)." So there was a narcotic, an addictive ingredient that caused both doctors to be critical in prescribing such a cough syrup. How cautious they were! But one thing she knew about herself that was 100 percent accurate, and that was her desire to steer clear of all illegal drugs. She was in all kinds of Just Say No" and D.A.R.E." clubs sponsored by the newspaper for young folks, and by golly, she even presented seminars on cocaine, pot, angel dust, ecstasy, meth, and the like. There was absolutely no way she was becoming addicted. She grew up in a Christian home, both parents stayed together with great respect for each other, Kym and her brother Spencer.

Kym and Spence always made fun of "druggies" on TV or in books, as the ones outlined in "People" Magazine like Kurt Cobain. Heck, they were stupid, funny, duh-h-h-hhh dumb. They were so much unlike the Corells that Kym couldn't believe young Cobain or River Phoenix hadn't gotten help to overcome their stupidity. "Their own fault; they deserved it!" she actually stated to her friends, who shook their clueless heads in agreement.

Two teaspoons left. What would be the best thing to do? Jiminy, I'm panicking, my heart is beating fast, and I am lost as to what I should do to become safely energized and fun-filled during the next several weeknights.

"I KNOW THIS ISN'T HURTING ME; IT'S NOT STREET DRUGS OR ANYTHING," she yelled into the mirror.

"I deserve this! Ryan has been too busy to spend much time with me lately, and work has been a bitch. I want to feel good and I will! I'm a darn good person and I'm not doing anything wrong!"

The problem was how to obtain more of the medicine without any problems, and she didn't know whether to contact another doctor or call Dr. York again. If she could convince him she was really in bad shape, or better yet—that she spilled the last bottle, but then it had taken several days to get spilled" and he would think she should be over the illness anyway. She decided to call Dr. Pirsky with the spill news" anyway, gulped once or twice, dialed the number and hung up three times before finally letting it ring, and swallowed hard. She was about to tell a white lie again. The first was to Dr. Pirsky about her horrible pneumonic infection, and the second now would be a false spilling of the bottle. She waited for Marlene to answer.

"Dr. Pirsky's office. Good morning!"

"Good morning, Marlene. It's Kymlin Corell."

"Hi, Kym! What's going on?"

"The uh, bottle of cough syrup Dr. Pirsky gave me was very much appreciated, but I dropped it on the floor before I could place the cap on, and it spilled. Could I have a refill just this once?"

Marlene noticed her heavy breathing on the other end, "Are you okay, Kym? You sound labored. Are you breathing better than you were when you came here?"

"Actually, the cough syrup is greatly missed. It was truly helping my nasty cough. Could you prescribe a couple of ounces to make up for the spilled stuff?"

"Just a minute."

Dr. P. came onto the phone. "What's the problem, Kymlin? You spilled some medicine?"

"Yes, I did. Since I'm still coughing, may I have a small refill?"

"I'm surprised you're not well yet. And wouldn't your syrup be gone by this time?"

"Well, yes—it was ALMOST gone, but the cough is still lingering."

"I can't give you more of the Tussionex, Kymlin. It's very addictive. We have those who called us regularly to report their meds stolen or spilled in hopes of getting more from me. Those patients have been terminated. Now, I don't think you're one of the addicted people who . . . "

"I understand, sir. I'll just wing it until it stops."

With that she hung up, a combination of panic and doom clouding her mind. It was time to go to an urgent care center.

Life is so amazing, because we plan it out with such precision and then—bingo! The least little footpath takes us into rough waters. Maybe if we realize when that footpath begins, when it starts to cause trouble, we could avoid all the consequences of moving down that footpath. But life has many twists and turns, leading us into bliss, happiness, sorrow and crisis. You never know when that road will offer the good and the bad, and when we should avoid that footpath entirely. Since we don't know the future, we are destined to take the footpath to find out what unexpectedly lay in store.

CHAPTER FOUR

Denial is a myriad of things, all of them meant to tell us lies. When we deny, we are setting ourselves up for untruths that will cost us in the long run. Denial is the ace repairman who promises a superb job but leaves a disaster behind. It is foolery unchained that causes the opposite of what we try to believe from happening. It is a one-way ticket to oblivion when we think we're grasping heaven. It is a "yes, yes" when reality says "no, no".

And so we go on our merry way, saying we're not addicted; we can stop anytime, but we simply enjoy getting high. Heck, take it away and we would adjust to the loss after a few days of lamenting.

And if we believe this, then there is lakefront property we can buy in Florida for one dollar a square mile.

No one purposely falls into the denial trap; it seems to pursue us to wield its ways. It's a ways and means committee that pushes, shoves, and even pleads for us to believe what it tells us. Problem is, it's all a lie, all sugar-coated and beckoning. And oh, is it ever believable! Convincingly it tells us that a crisis isn't even a minor dilemma, that we can handle it, take care of it, squelch it if need be.

It won't ever baffle us, because we have the answers. Of course we're not addicts; addicts are street people who grasp at a fix constantly from the local drug dealer who would just as soon blow us away.

Addicts are never medicine junkies. Medicines heal, they are prescribed, they are good for us, they minimize the pain. Question is: Which pain do they heal? Is it the legitimate post-surgical or injury pain that they help? Or is it the pain of fear, of that withdrawal that seems a hundred times greater than any flu bug? Doesn't this prove that a medicine junkie is still a junkie?

If you asked Kimlyn Corell, she would tell you at this time how much she has her head on straight, how little she actually needs (she would say "uses"), and if anyone asked her to quit, she would ponder about pursuing it. Not pursue it, just PONDER about pursuing it. You see, it's up to her, not the fates. She just wants another day or two so she can easily wean off the pain meds.

But Kimlyn is just about to enter the "denial zone", and she will be surprised by what she finds there. For no matter how much she minimizes her dependence (oops—we mean "use"), she is hooked on narcotics. She can promise every friend, family member, work associate, and minister that she'll pitch the meds out this week, but deep down in the abyss of her mind a struggle is going on. This abyss is not in denial; it holds the truth. That reality tells Kimlyn's subconscious that she would rather give up her left arm than her narcotics. Her conscious mind remains naïve, and so she will continue to deny the boulder-size problem until her subconscious and conscious mind agree that "something's got to give".

We can only hope she grasps reality before jail, legal problems, ill health or even death becomes reality too.

Will she or won't she be saved from herself? Can she look ahead to the mountain of problems and GPS right to her subconscious, where the truth awaits?

We can only hope and pray to the God she needs to renew in her life. In the meantime, Kimlyn's story continues . . . .

CHAPTER FIVE

There was just such a center about two miles from her home, and she'd heard the doctor is a generous prescriber of many meds. Now she would find out if her desired med was one he would give her.

The wait was phenomenally long because everyone could just walk right in, sign up, and sit. She had 14 patients ahead of her this day. When she was called up to the desk to fill out papers and insurance info, she mustered up a sigh of relief, thinking she had been called to come back and be seen. No such luck.

The afternoon was shot, and evening was fast approaching. It was nice to be on a 7:30 a.m. to 3:30 p.m. schedule, but it would be nearly 6:30 before she could be seen, she guessed.

Finally, her turn came, and she literally jumped up from the soft brown davenport to go on back. Her nurse was a well-scrubbed young girl named "Elle," who told her the doctor she was to see was Dr. Worley, a woman. She pleasantly said thank you and was left in the examining room for about five minutes after vitals were taken by Elle.

In walked Dr. Talina Worley, an attractive woman of about 40. She inquired about the problem facing Kym today.

Kym was well-rehearsed now. She exclaimed that the cough was making her very weary, may be serious, and may be pneumonia.

Dr. Worley proceeded to cut her off before she could say any more.

"Let me be the judge of what is ailing you, honey. We'll give it a good try."

After answering a series of unwanted questions, Dr. Worley agreed that the cough sounded pretty serious and needed a suppressant rather than a decongestant. Her choice was not welcome to Kym. It was a non-narcotic that was sold over the counter called Claritin. Kym tried to barter with her but it was to no avail; this doctor was sharp as a tack, and with a walk-in practice she was particularly wary of drug-seekers.

Dejected and disappointed, she made her way to the car, panicking while depression took its toll over the next hour. The last doctor she intended to see was the one to whom her mother went prior to finding Dr. York. His name was Dr. Murray Stascheck, and he was of the old school and bedside manner. She reasoned that the only reason Mom began to see Dr. York was because she wanted to team up York and Kym, which of course was like pairing water and oil, she thought,. She was extrovert and enjoyed being the center of attention, unlike York, who was introvert extraordinaire.

Stascheck was indeed a super-nice guy, and invited Kym as if she were the Queen of Sheba into his examining room. But then everything became unraveled. His methods were of the old school and included narcotics only rarely, and not for bronchitis, he told her. Then she had her first insult (or so she viewed it) from a physician:

"Young Lady, if you expect to get narcotics for your ailment, you've come to the wrong physician. I want to help patients, not addict them."

The nerve of that man! No wonder Mom went to York now. "He practically called me a drug addict!" she fumed to herself.

To make a long chapter short, Kymlin Corell ended up visiting over 120 physicians in seven counties to obtain Tussionex or a similar cough syrup with hydrocodone called Hycodan and Vicodin-Tuss. By this time in 1990, she was 40 years old, addicted to the point of making cough syrup the No. 1 priority in her life, and yet she hadn't even really gotten "wet behind the ears" in addiction. She hadn't gone to rehabs, prison, blown a marriage and almost two of them, or come to know what could literally save her life. All these and more experiences were going to hit hard in the near future, because she was becoming infamous and well-known to the Akron Police Department and other lawmen. Kym had no idea what lay in store. One of the hardships was about to enthrall her for the seventh time: severe withdrawal from narcotics. It was the lesser of all the hardships to come, but it wasn't pretty either. Had she stopped at two teaspoons, withdrawal would have been minimal. However, over the next couple of years she had advanced to at least six spoonfuls, and once in a while endured ten. It could all have been avoided, for many of the physicians she visited told her the truth about drugs and about what was happening to her on them. Do addicts in progression ever listen? Rarely, until they hit bottom.

And this is just one stop toward that descent: WITHDRAWAL.

CHAPTER SIX

The first day she failed to get her fix wasn't as bad as the next three days. The thought never left her: If only I had gone to that other doctor . . . . But she hadn't. And now she was in for a myriad of awful symptoms until she could drag herself to a doctor who would take her present symptoms mistakenly for flu or bronchitis. That would be the ploy. Was it going to work?

She had pretty much exhausted the various physicians in her realm of travel, especially the way she felt presently. No one should drive in the condition she found herself a day and a half after her last dose. So she decided to tough it out, but only while calling around until she could make an appointment for a visit to one of the dozens of doctors she had visited in the past few years. Oh, she had heard it all by now: grooming for an addictive lifestyle, said one; many had gone on their computers and found her name came up as a patient to avoid because of what she was seeking from them. Still others called her a liar and told her to get out of their offices, which was most embarrassing. Yes, she had heard it all, and yet she didn't care because she would give her left leg to be able to find a compassionate doctor who would give her just a couple of ounces to ward off the demons for at least one more day.

The first day she felt rotten, but not half-dead. She had chills and headaches, but not much more beyond those symptoms. The second day was a different story.

All hell broke loose. Besides the chills and headaches, about fifteen new symptoms bombarded her aching, withdrawing body. First, the chills and headaches kicked in early—very early—in the a.m., followed by diarrhea, vomiting, and restless leg syndrome. Then she felt antsy, depressed, helpless, and restless all over. She could not sit still. She paced back and forth from the hall to her bedroom, over and over, at least 100 times, then began to cry. This was day three, the worst of the lot.

She HAD to find a prescribing doctor, she HAD to. It was 3:00 Friday afternoon, and the doctors would mostly have called it a short day, unfortunately. So she thought she'd just tough it out until something happened, even if it meant enduring Saturday and Sunday. She would do it. Much as she dreaded it, she would have to do it. Then Monday would follow, and she could look for someone new, again. What a life this had become. She had no other priorities, but if this one could be satisfied, that's all that mattered, and she would then be able to carry out her work better, and household duties. Fortunately this was spring break/vacation she had put in for, and that's the only aspect that enabled her to keep her job during this bout with multiple symptoms, about five times worse than those the flu would produce.

She had hoped to enjoy her vacation with her little plastic, gold-filled friend, but it didn't happen that way. These symptoms were some of the worst she'd ever experienced, even when she had the flu. She was bed-bound completely, except going to the bathroom (diarrhea) or trying to force something down, eating some little thing just so she'd not feel hunger pangs along with all the other symptoms. But it was perfectly miserable, and she cried a lot.

She didn't feel like calling any friends or relatives, watching TV, or anything else she usually did when bedridden, because she couldn't concentrate on anything except her illness. She thought if she called one of the many physicians she had called previously, perhaps he or she would come through, and once again Kym would enjoy her bottle. But she had run out of refill requests from every doctor who would give them until they said no, and all she could do was think of someone she hadn't gone to yet. She would put on a stiff upper lip and try to control the way she felt just until she could overcome her quivering voice for a few minutes. Unfortunately, when she perused the phone book, almost everyone under family practice or internal medicine or even general practice had been seen to the max or she would have to have a physical before they would examine anything else, and that would be another visit since she was a new patient. She growled under her breath.

Toughing it out was the only alternative, and she was already halfway through it, almost three days. Bottom really had to be hit before any let-up and crawling up the mountain could be achieved. So, bear it she did—reluctantly.

She yearned for a bottle of golden goo worse than anything she ever desired, even a date with a classy new beau earlier. She knew this because she was to marry Ryan sometime in the near future, she had told him, and now she didn't even think of him one-tenth as much as the bottle of cough syrup. Ryan couldn't even compare with a lousy container of addictive syrup. That was pretty sad, she thought.

Concentration was the most difficult thing to do now, more difficult than she could ever imagine in the past. But she counted the minutes and realized in one more day there was one refill available she overlooked in her misery. One refill—she'd pay over $100 for it if she had the money this week. She hadn't even gone to the bank to cash her paycheck or pay bills. Nothing else mattered, nothing, nothing. Just a couple of ounces of Tussionex or Hycodan would do the trick and alleviate this horrible withdrawal, and hallelujah—it would be available tomorrow. If only she could get through today . . . .

She did. And at precisely 9:00 a.m. she was on her way to MedAm Pharmacy. Even though Dr. Pirsky had frowned on refills, he made a MISTAKE and actually issued one. It said one refill, his mistake, but Kym thought was a blessing. She was ecstatic.

Of course it didn't last for more than a few hours, because two ounces translates to 12 teaspoons, and she was not frugal with the dosage. Then it was back to square one. Wait! She was told about a pain management doctor by Marla at work a few weeks ago, and she had the phone number. Would she be off and rolling? Could he see her tomorrow—or even what was left of today? She doubted the latter, but she called as quickly as she could.

"Good afternoon. Dr. Sigor's office. May we help you?"

"I . . . I hope so. My name is Kymlin Corell, and I've had some terrific pain in my legs, probably fibromyalgia, according to my regular doctor."

He wanted her to see Dr. Sigor, she lied.

"Could you come in next week? Say, about Tuesday or Wednesday, around 1:00? He's really double-booked until then."

"Uh, yes, but I'm really in misery. I would only take up a few minutes of your time, really, but do you think you'll have any cancellations?"

"Oh, we have a few from time to time. And just fifteen minutes ago one came in for 2:00 tomorrow. But I had to place a gentleman in that spot. First come, first served. You understand, don't you?"

"Could you double-book me with him, just this once? I'm willing to wait, really. Please, could you . . . "

The receptionist interrupted her.

"Kymlin, I'm sorry; that would not be possible. This gentleman IS double-booked with someone else. You are a new patient, too, so you would need a physical first. That's a complication I'd almost forgotten about. I'm really sorry."

Kym hung up without even telling her goodbye, which was something she NEVER did with anyone—even wrong numbers. She was pissed.

Pissed!

Kym made it through, and on day four she washed up and bathed, shampooed her hair, brushed her teeth, and did all the little things she had neglected due to her insistence to get the medicine in the throes of withdrawal. Three days later, she was through withdrawal, but she still desired that delicious euphoric optimism. This continued even throughout the first months of her marriage, which was Sept. 22, 1990. She was now 40, and wondered if life would begin for her. She had quit the newspaper because Ryan lived about 60 miles away, and tried to get a job in Youngstown, where she now lived. But she sabotaged herself with tardiness, absenteeism, illness, and drug addiction that were beginning to be discovered.

Once her purse fell and everything fell from it, including a small bottle of the Tussionex, which she had to work really hard to obtain. Remember—120 doctors in these last few years is quite a number. Her co-worker Charles, a goof in his own right, made fun of the bottle as it rolled onto the floor. He pretended she was boozing, and spread the word. Angry as she was, she knew addiction had claimed her in some sordid ways, and she didn't refute his accusations, just told him to MYOB!

Ryan was the first to discover her dependency. He even told her he'd help her in any way he could, all she had to do was tell him how to deal with it. The wall remained between them, though, and Ryan grew more and more dissatisfied with the doctor bills and bottles that came into his home.

"Kymmi, I think you are an addict. There, I said it, and I'm sorry to hurt you, but the truth hurts, honey."

"Thanks a heap, Mr. Tact! You know I can take it or leave it if I really, really have to do it. It's just been hard at work lately with all the holiday ads they're throwing at us, and I need something to feel good about when I get home."

"I'm not good enough for you? Do you really need that yellow crap? We're newlyweds, and I thought just the two of us would be a good team. But I've got competition from a stupid six-inch tall bottle and its goopy contents. We've been married only a few months and I've got competition. I could handle another man, sweetie, but I can't handle this stuff."

'Oh, come on, Ryan~ It's only medicine that helps my mood. I . . ." She was cut short.

"Honey, I got a call today from the Sheriff's office. They want you to come in tomorrow morning to talk about your medicine."

"What? What about it? I'm legal, I'm going through doctors and not going to any street corner for REAL drugs; I'm too smart for that. What does the man want?"

"He's a lieutenant, Gaines is his name, I think. I don't think you'll be arrested or anything like that, but . . . "

"Arrested?—*Arrested*! What did you tell him?"

"Not much; he really wants to speak with you tomorrow. Look, baby, I don't think it's anything serious, but you have been going to scads of physicians, and our medical insurance is complaining. Just, please, talk to him."

Without fully realizing her addiction had begun to claim her legally, she was worried about the possibility that she could ever be arrested. She was a clean-living, moral person who just happened to relish cough syrup. Why did they want to take it away from her—if that was what this would be about.

CHAPTER SEVEN

Kym arrived at the police station about 10 a.m. the next day, noticeably flustered and somewhat belligerent-appearing. She slammed down her purse on a nearby chair and ignored everyone who came close to her. Lt. Gaines, a rather formidable-looking gentleman with sandy hair and a mustache, approached her and introduced himself, requesting that they go into a quieter, smaller room to speak.

"Yeah, I guess so, okay," she replied. "Just what is this all about, Lieutenant? Have I done something HORRIBLY wrong?" she asked, sarcastic on purpose.

"Mrs. Danzen, you have crossed the law by going to so many doctors for what appears to be a narcotic addiction. The term for this felony is called "Deception to obtain a dangerous drug" and it can carry up to three years in prison. Have you anything to say about your . . . . problem?"

"I didn't go to anyone but doctors, Lieutenant Gaines. And . . . FELONY? What is this all about? How can it be something illegal? I hid nothing from anyone."

"Kymlin, that is not quite true. Of the 34 doctors I've spoken to, several said they did not know you had just visited another doctor prior to your visit with then, That makes it dishonest and illegal, especially when we're talking about narcotics. People will do a lot to get high on codeine-type derivatives."

Now she understood. She was playing with fire, and the computer system could easily trace her prescriptions from one place to another. Oh, no . . . she was cooked. Her life was over. Until Lt. Gaines told her:

"You have never been in trouble with the law before, Mrs. Danzen. This is just a warning that you cannot continue to practice doctor-shopping, as it is called on the street. Do you read me?"

"Yes, I do. May I be excused now? I understand and it won't happen again."

Somehow when she promised him it wouldn't occur any longer, she was not dedicated to the idea of ceasing her doctor-shopping. There is no way she would end up in jail for seeing a bunch of doctors. Screw Gaines.

He dismissed her with an admonition:

"Please, Mrs. Danzen, please note that you could end up in jail, or even prison if you need one very soon, like NOW. Will you promise me you'll seek treatment?"

"Yeah, sure. If you think it would help me," she answered half-heartedly.

"I do, but you'd better not wait too long. Your marriage could break up, you could spend a few years in prison, your life could be ruined if you hesitate. I know a very good clinic in northern Youngstown called The Clinic for Narcotic and Drinking Help" that I think would be ideal for your rehab, but you and your husband will need to talk it over. Goodbye now, and good luck."

Her head was spinning when he left. Prison? Divorce? Life in ruins?

C'mon, I'm NOT a problem to anyone except myself, and I like getting euphoric—or high, or whatever, just at night. This guy is coming on like gangbusters just too scare me. Prison is for criminals, felons, and . . . Oh, he said I was a felon, didn't he?

Well, there's no way a misdemeanor should be termed a felony. That guy can go jump off a bridge; I'm not quitting."

When she arrived home, she and Ryan talked over what Lt. Gaines had said to her. Ryan was wholeheartedly in favor of the rehab. The cost of CNDH was $20,000 and insurance would pay, which made Ryan quite happy, while Kym just continued be to melancholy. She did not want to give up her golden sunshine of a syrup, even no one else could see he value in it.

There were heavy disagreements, discussions, and finally, with the promise that if it didn't work she could go back to at least a week's worth of Tussionex, she agreed to go.

CHAPTER EIGHT

She really didn't want to quit, deep down, because she enjoyed that feeling the narcotic provided. Still, she didn't want to irk the law any more than she already had, so she agreed to go into that stupid place. One thing she couldn't shake, the one thing that probably pushed her more than anything else, was her father's death in July. It was August now, but her father turned to her mom in the hospital before he died from Lou Gehrig's disease and begged, "Chrissy, please get Kymlin off that cough syrup." Then he died.

Her parents did not live very far away, so they kept tabs on Kym as if they lived in the same house, especially after she caught this habit. Her brother Spence was a recovering alcoholic and was doing beautifully, but he had attended a LOT of Alcoholics Anonymous meetings and other 12-step groups.

Kym still didn't believe she had a problem, at least not one she couldn't solve. But she was in denial greatly. Kym's mom helped her pack for the clinic with the admonition that if she came back home still clinging to that bottle she would exit Kym's life for good. The habit had taken a terrific toll on her family, especially after her father's slow death. Christine Corell did not have the patience of Job.

Ryan had a lot more patience, but he, too, had become discouraged upon finding a huge paper bag with at least 20 bottles that had once contained Tussionex in a drawer of Kym's dresser. He was overjoyed that she agreed to go to the rehab.

That afternoon, Wednesday, Kym's car with Ryan driving went to a place Kym would never have made her destination without much prodding: The Clinic.

A couple of young men came out to the car to help her bring in her suitcase and other belongings; after all, this was to be a 35-day stint, not just withdrawal and detox from withdrawal. Before she went inside, Ryan asked to see her purse. She balked, saying that it was her own personal property and he didn't have to worry, but he lost patience and snatched it. Inside was a bottle containing at least four ounces of syrup. He confiscated it, and she put up a big stink.

"Ryan, that is mine. I got it from my doctor."

"No, it is not yours. This is what you are coming here to get rid of. I'm really surprised you'd do this. So you want to get well by being sue you had a bottle. What? You wanted to enjoy the activities and have no sweat off your back? Sorry, Kym, it ends here."

She threatened to go back home, but Ryan would have none of it. He told her she would have no home to come back to if she didn't stick out the program for a month. When she saw several welcoming faces, she decided to go on in. But what a struggle! She almost decked Ryan in the process of "Whose bottle is it?"

For the next 35 days she played the game: volleyball, songs, meditations, talent shows, prayer and AA meetings, and much, much more. It was a fine clinic, privately owned, but nevertheless intent on helping those who entered there. If they wanted it, that is.

What Kym didn't tell anyone is that she had a refill coming due about week three of the stint in CDNH. She even used the unmonitored telephone to check on the status of the bottle before she was released. Yes, it would be there for her pick-up soon.

She shared a dorm room with a small woman about 55 named Elyse. One evening the two were talking and Elyse offered a nutshell of her personal failures due to a years-long bout with cocaine.

"Hey, Kym, don't go out of here without learning something. It's a privilege for me to be here instead of in prison."

"Prison? What did you do that would have sent you to prison?"

"Dear, you're wet behind the ears; I bet this is your first rehab. Yes, I ended up in the slammer because I was dealing cocaine."

"I never dealt anything. I went to doctors. I would never deal."

"That's what they all say, until you're forced into a very bad situation. I had two kids by the time I was fifteen, and their dad abandoned me. I had no income, and the only way I could make ends meet then with no GED or diploma was to deal coke. But I got into trouble plenty, and went to prison after a drug bust. Oh, yeah—there was a shootout at my friend's house (he was dealing too) and two customers got killed. I did two years just for being at the wrong place at the wrong time."

"Don't say you ain't ever done this or that, because there is a big YET at the end of every sentence," warned Elle.

"Look, Elle, I know your life is a lot different than mine, because of all you went through. And I'm sorry you had to endure all that. But all I did was get euphoric on a little cough syrup, which I wish I had right now," Kym confessed. "Especially since I feel like hell without it. Oh, sure, the valiums they give help a little, but . . . . ."

"You're in denial, Kym. Big time. I never want to see another white powder of any kind again. I guess you haven't reached bottom yet."

"No, I guess it's just the pits for me, so the bottom is still waiting, and I don't care. I sure would drink the stuff if I had it on me."

"I feel sorry for you, Kym. You don't know anything about what they're trying to do for you here. Until you do, you'll never get better. You'll be dry' until they can get through to you. You don't want to go to prison, do you? I tell you, it's hopeless there. I did a decade and I will do anything to keep from going there again, If you knew what it was like, you would avoid it any way you could. Dry isn't sober. It's just white-knuckling it until your next fix. Give it up, Kym. Don't hang on to something that hurts you, Why don't you come to the AA meeting this afternoon? You'll see how the tools work. I haven't had cocaine now for two weeks, and I'm glad, I can't guarantee forever, just one day at a time, but at least now I'll have a life. You can too. And that man at home—do it for him, too. Ryan sounds like an okay guy."

"He is, yes. But I think he makes a big deal out of this cough syrup."

"Didn't you say the police became involved with your case? That isn't real insignificant."

"Oh, they just didn't have anyone else to pick on that day. It's okay. I really don't need this place to so-called get well. I can quit if I try real hard, on my own."

"That's what I said too. But it took loss of life and prison to make me realize I needed help. And I still do. That's why I'm here, Kym. I still need help. They counsel you, play kinda silly games, show movies, and much more. You'll grow to like it if you just try. Otherwise, your life isn't going to be worth a plugged nickel."

"Look, Elle, I wish you would mind your own business, okay? It might have been that way for you but it isn't for me. So just—can it."

"Okay. It's your problem, your death sentence, not mine. But I tried to tell you. Someday you'll remember me."

"Yeah, you're right. MY life, not yours."

Elle gave her a pathetic-eye look and turned around, walked away down the hall. But, like so many others now (relatives not excluded), Kym was on many people's minds. She was salvageable, but did she want to be saved, or just to continue in her blindness and limited euphoria?

As the days came and went, the pleasant but demanding program took its tiring toll on the clients, and by midnight they were ready to drop from exhaustion. But many thought it challenging and worth the work. These are the people who would make it, who understood what they were up against. Kym still didn't fathom her formidable foe. That refill still beckoned her, and in only three days her 35 would be up. Then she could have her optimism back.

The last day saw many tearful goodbyes. Kym had made several friends, but she never melted, and everyone knew her sobriety was not going to last. Not once did she admit she was in the throes of an addiction; not once did she cry when mentioning Lt. Gaines. Her rhetoric seemed almost rehearsed, and it was evident that she spoke only to fulfill the requirements of the program. She couldn't wait for 1:00 to come, because then Ryan would pick her up and she could go out later to pick up her refill. He would never know; she was just going to visit one of the girls from the rehab."

CHAPTER NINE

She was to go to an AA meeting near the drugstore where her refill was located, so while the 12 Steps were being read she had already picked up her bottle and dosed 10 teaspoons. That little plastic spoon in the dish drainer was perfect to smuggle in her purse. She suddenly realized just how profound those steps sounded, just like the pleasure derived from doing that crossword puzzle when she first took two teaspoonfuls. Then she sobered up rather quickly, even if for just a moment. It took two teaspoons to achieve the same effect—perhaps even stronger than now—and this was five times as many spoons as on that first, fateful day. Her tolerance had grown, a least that is what the rehab would have responded had she told anyone there of her increase.

The rest of the meeting was okay, even enjoyable, but in the back of her mind she pondered that ten spoons was the equivalent of almost two ounces at once. What was happening to her? But she knew. She knew.

Unfortunately her life during the next three years was made up of several rehabs, very much the same as the one she first visited, and Ryan's patience was growing less and less tolerant. Finally she came across a rehab that seemed as if it would work, and she vowed to stay clean. But there was a reason for this, it wasn't just because she didn't want to use any more. That reason was Barry Felden. Ryan finally called off the living together marriage, and thought since Kym was heading into a three-month inpatient rehab center, he would see how things went when she came to her senses—if she would. But he no longer wanted her under the same roof until she could prove herself and kick the syrup. In other words, they were separated, not just by Hilton Harvester Rehab, but she would have to find another place to stay when she was clean again.

Barry was a client who looked like David Hasselhoff of Baywatch, but he was rather slow on the draw following a near-fatal auto accident. Still, he paid her special attention from Day One, and she, at 45, was flattered. He was only 38 but had trouble with cocaine and was in this, his third rehab. Kym had completed four detoxes and three in-patient rehabs before Harvester, and nothing had clocked until now. Why? Because she had a new face to deal with.

Ryan had gained custody of his psychotic, hyperactive six-year-old son, and this thrown into the mix was driving her crazy at home. Ryan lived for the little brat, and she always ranked a far second. With her newfound vulnerability, she was actually looking around for someone new. Had she been sober, she probably could have handled the situation much more easily or with greater finesse, but she was a flop as a step-parent.

One thing she was not a flop at was greeting the public. Harvester was having a corporate meeting day in which one of the clients would be telling his/her story to many leaders of Akron, just to educate them to addiction and the toll it had taken on their life. Even though Kym couldn't see the forest for the trees, she could fortify her speech with memorable terms, even though she didn't feel she had hit bottom yet. Still, she would do her best, because Barry would be proud of her.

She also was invited by the Akron newspaper to tell her story, and how addiction had left her with much less than she had before. Unfortunately, she could talk, talk, talk, but she didn't feel this great loss just yet. But she wanted to be in the limelight. Maybe she could help someone who REALLY needed a story like that to examine. Might make them feel better.

The story came out on a 225,000 circulation day and was entitled, HOOKED'. Front page, she didn't expect that. Good thing she had decided she wanted Barry more than drugs. She knew she was in for some criticism and surprise expressions from those who knew her—even her close relatives. She never thought it would be in the Sunday edition with the highest readership of the week.

She hadn't lost nearly as much as most folks in addiction have. Just part of her marriage and some family criticism and—oh, yes, her esteem from that pesky Lt. Gaines. But now she was a local celebrity, which was not going to go down well with her judge when she exited the rehab. Something else had happened.

Kym had been prescribed naltrexone to dampen cravings for opiates; in fact, if it were used at the same time as this medicine, not one ion of euphoria would be noticeable. The molecules would stay on the receptors in the brain and remain sticky enough to send the opiate molecules packing. They could not break through the "pleasure pathway" as this part of the brain was deemed. Neurons were doomed to failure when any hint of euphoria tried to make an entrance. It just wouldn't happen. She had been issued the naltrexone about three weeks earlier, and the cravings were nil. She really missed that euphoria, that "feeling", but she could pick it up anytime later. There were several more doctors now in practice in northeast Ohio.

Right now Barry made her high. They simply joked, ate together, sang, did karaoke, worked together on Harvester projects, and the like. She just didn't need drugs right now. She had Barry.

Then she realized what Barry's problem had been: He was more than a bit shaken up by that awful auto accident. He was mentally challenged to the hilt. Real brawn, no brains, she thought. And he was playing up to the younger female clients. Oh, well.

"Kym, I have a message for you, and it doesn't sound happy," said Darwyn Sellers, one of the clients.

"What? What is it?" asked Kym.

"I'm supposed to tell you that Judge Cooley will see you in her chambers tomorrow morning at 9 a.m. Don't know what it's about. They wouldn't tell me."

Why in the world would a judge ask to see her? She was in a rehab; she was where she supposed to should be. Maybe if she talked to Shayla, her counselor . . . Yes! Shay would reason with her and be honest as to what she knows. So to Shayla she went.

"Surprised" was not the word she thought. Horror was more appropriate.

"Shayla, why does Judge Cooley want to see me tomorrow? Do you know?"

Suddenly the atmosphere was theatrical, unreal, or surreal. Shayla told her, "YOU are going to Ohio Penitentiary for Women after what you did!"

Kym was dumbfounded. What did she do? How could she be sent to prison? She had to find out more; she was hysterical.

She ran to the administrator's office. Max Devine was a super nice gentleman and was the one who chose Kym for the corporate Akron talks last week. If anyone could help, he could.

"Max, Max! Is it true I'm going to OPW? What on earth did I do? Huh? What are you trying to do to me? I'm clean and I haven't cheated!"

The bespectacled tall, gaunt leader looked her in the eye.

"Kymlin, your urine was positive for alcohol. We know that's an ingredient in Tussionex. You've broken our stringent rules about specimens, and after four rehabs, you've had it, lady! Why did you do it?"

She was sobbing wildly now.

"But I didn't! I've been clean since I came here because I knew there could be a life for me after all these years! I'm not stupid enough to put that on the line! You tell that judge . . . . "

"Tell her yourself. You've got to be in her chambers at 8:30 tomorrow morning."

She began packing her clothes to go to her mother's, for she agreed to house Kym until she found a room or apartment. She was asked what she was doing by Elle.

"Kym, why are you packing? You have a few more days yet."

"No, I don't. I've just been told I'm going to prison for a bad urine when I haven't had Tussionex or alcohol or hydrocodone since before I came to this blasted place. Something is very wrong. Someone has got the samples mixed up! I don't drink and there is no alcohol in Tussionex anyway! Elle, what am I going to do?"

"Come on to my room and we'll talk. It can't be that bad."

But Kym knew it was that bad, even the worst. But why was another story.

"Kim, what exactly happened?" Elle asked Kym when they were both sitting on her bunk bed.

"I was doing fine, I thought. I put on a talent show, did projects, and all that was required. I NEVER used Tussionex or any other illegal drug while I've been here. Now I'm told by Max and Shayla that I'm on my way to prison for bad urine, which couldn't happen because I've been clean for weeks! Elle, what's happening to me?" she nearly screamed.

:You've got to calm down. You're hyperventilating. Do you want me to talk with them?"

"You won't get any further than I did. They seemed surreal, almost as if what they had to say was part of a play. Their attitude toward me was nearly hostile. I can't understand what has really happened."

"Are you sure you didn't slip once or twice? It's easy to do."

"Not for me, not now. No, I was proud of my record because it made me look more heroic in front of Barry. But I did it for myself too."

"I'll see what I can do, chickie. Hang tough!"

"Okay, okay. I'll see who else I can talk to, but maybe they were just trying to scare me. I'll try talking to that new nurse, Crystal. Wish me luck, Elle. Please!"

"You got it, kid! Go get 'em!"

Before Kym was fully packed, she asked to speak with Crystal, and was told she was a bit busy at the moment. But in a few, she could see me for a couple of minutes. And over she came just a minute later.

"Hi, Kym. What's up?"

"I think I'm going to prison tomorrow. I've got to talk with Judge Cooley, but before that I've got to speak to someone here who knows what's going on."

Crystal seemed surprised.

"What's the problem? You didn't beat up on anyone, kill someone, steal drugs, or anything like that at all. In fact, your urines have been clean since you entered Harvesters. What's the deal here?"

"That's just it, I don't know! Right now the only thing that will help me is prayer."

"How do they know Judge Cooley is going to imprison you?"

Kym was silent, shrugged her shoulders, and started to cry again. They knew something she didn't, and it wasn't fair. She hadn't even been heard yet. This was supposed to be a rehab that ended with her victory over drugs and she could have her life back. And maybe Barry's too. Now she didn't know what was happening and who was carrying out this plan.

That evening she told her mother what had happened as she unpacked her bags, and her mother started to cry.

"Why did you use, Kym? Why??"

Kym began to cry when she saw her mother did not believe her honesty. Barry was still at the rehab and she realized he was at the back of her mind now in comparison with what was facing her, and how everyone knew she was going to prison before she had even heard the news.

"What did you do, Kymmi? How stupid could you be when you were in that plush rehab? You know, you stole those antique dishes from me a few years ago to support your habit, and those hand-painted dishes were worth at least $200. You went to a doctor, got your prescription, and paid for it with the money you got at the antique shop. I know, I know. Maxine works there, and she told me."

Who was Maxine? Oh, well, time to call some people to find out what to do. There as only nighttime now, then . . . . oh, Dear Jesus!

She had to get in touch with her family lawyer, Jim Gorner, She could call him at home; he must be getting ready for tomorrow morning. Why didn't he call me? Surely he knew I was going to court. Oh well, here goes . . . .

She dialed, and Jim answered immediately.

"Hello, Gorner here. What can I do for you?"

"Atty. Gorner, this is Kymlin Corell. Obviously you knew what happened today, I'm supposed to see Judge Cooley tomorrow at 8:30 a.m.

I don't understand because I've complied with all the rules in the rehab. You know, I called you before I went into the place. But why am I seeing her? Everyone at the rehab tells me I am heading for OPW. But I didn't have any bad urines! They say I did! What do I do, Mr. Gorner?"

"What are you talking about, Kym? You know if you were to see the judge I would be there to represent you. I have had no calls about this at all, I think you're mistaken, but if they told you what time to be there, I suppose I'd better go, in case something is up. Now, you're telling me you're being accused of having dirty urine when in fact this did not happen?"

"Yes, sir. I've done nothing wrong. I am on naltrexone which negates any effects of an opiate like the one I had taken previously, hydrocodone, and so there would be no reason to take any opiate. Plus I am finally happy with what I'm doing. I was in denial, they say, about my drug use but now I understand what that means. Atty. Gorner, I'm no dummy. Can you help me?"

He sighed.

"I just don't understand why I was not contacted about this hearing. But I will be there, Kym, and we'll try to straighten all this out."

"Thank you, sir. Oh, yes—they say there is alcohol in my urine, and I'm allergic to drinking alcohol. I know there is no alcohol in Tussionex, even if I had taken it. So you see, nothing makes sense here."

"Yes, I see why you're flustered. Just be there at 8:30 and we'll see what goes down, er, happens. Sorry."

"That's okay. Oh, yes—they want to transport me there—the rehab. They apparently don't trust me to do it on my own,"

"Okay, Kym. See you at 8:30."

"Thanks so much—I really mean that."

"Your case is my case, honey. We'll see what's up."

She felt a sense of relief when she hung up. Perhaps nothing much was going to happen since her attorney hadn't even been told about the hearing. She would try to get a good night's sleep at her mother's, then go on down to the courthouse with Harvester transport. She was beginning to feel relieved, because she knew Gorner would do everything in his power to show the court how sober she is, and she would probably cry spontaneously as she so often did lately, but she would fight for her freedom, if worse came to worse.

CHAPTER TEN

Harvester came at 7:15 a.m., and she was ready. She had just combed her hair and finished her makeup. She felt a sense of triumph somehow, but she did not want to get her hopes up too far yet. Then she was there. She walked into the courthouse with one of the Harvester r counselors whose ear she had bent all the way during the half-hour drive. The counselor merely listened and grunted most of the time.

She sat down on the bench outside the judge's chambers. Atty. Gorner was there—bless him. Suddenly at 8:30 sharp he was beckoned into Judge Cooley's courtroom, while Kym sat outside. What was going on here? Why hadn't they called her in?

She fidgeted for nearly an hour, when suddenly Gorner came out of the courtroom. This was not going to be a picnic, according to his facial expression, which was drawn and scowling.

"Kym, she says you had Tussionex with alcohol, and a large amount appeared in your urine."

"I didn't! Please, let me see her."

"She didn't want to. She called you a newshound because of the story you co-wrote in the Akron newspaper, and said you love publicity. She is sentencing you to four years in Johnsburg, at OPW. I don't know why this is so trumped up or why I wasn't called but she has the say-so right now."

"But that can't be my urine. Did she check for naltrexone? That would prove I haven't had any opiates with any alcohol in them. She couldn't have found hydrocodone because damn it, I never used!"

She was telling the truth to thin air. No one was listening. Her escort driver just looked at her and sighed, "I don't know, Kym."

Gorner interrupted their non-chat.

"Kym, I'll look into this further. But it looks like you're going to have to do some time at OPW. She didn't even want to SEE you. Apparently she dislikes you from the newspaper article, and thought it was a plea that multiple rehabs should be tried before an addict is sent to prison. She is really hard-nosed, Kym. The article was good, but the judge thinks that in case it ever came down to this, your ulterior motive was to avoid prison."

"I hadn't even been approached by anything resembling the threat of prison, until yesterday. Bad timing on the article, you're telling me?"

"I guess so. Kym, someone is beckoning for you to follow her. I think you're going to be on transport to County Jail for now. And by the way, did you by any chance have a small bottle of Tussionex on you, perhaps in your purse?"

"Oh, no! With the depth of my black hole called a purse I've carried it for weeks, just as a security blanket, I guess. But I never used it."

"I believe you but the judge doesn't. Your purse was rummaged yesterday before you left the rehab."

"What? If anyone had the notion to go into my purse, they'd see that it was still full after all this time, and why would they do that anyway? Isn't that illegal?"

"Not when you're in a rehab facility. I'm surprised they didn't tell you to open your purse and spill the contents to them."

"No, they never did. But someone had an eye on it, I guess. Maybe a counselor. No money was missing, nothing was missing. I never dreamed someone would go through my purse at a well-guarded rehab like Harvesters."

"As I said, they can do that as long as you are in the facility. And this is not good for you, because they found the cough syrup that you are supposed to be off all this time. I believe you were, but they wouldn't even check it, said the judge. She saw the bottle, and that was enough, plus the urine . . . . "

"That could not have been my urine, I tell you. There would have been hydrocodone and instead there was naltrexone. Why would I take an opiate when I know it wouldn't do a bit of good?"

"Got me, Kym. Listen try to tough it out for a few months, then I'll try to get you out on shock probation. You would be on probation for perhaps three years, but you would not be in any facility. You could live with your mom or find a place of your own. You would have to report to a probation officer every week or two, but there would be no prison or jail. I will try to do this, but it will take up to three months."

Three months in prison before anything could be attempted to spring her. Why? Will anyone listen to her story about naltrexone, or what? Things may have gone differently if the judge weren't on the Harvesters Board of Administrators, but she now knew she'd been framed for something she didn't do. Just when she was getting straight, she would be thrust into OPW. She had done the story on rehab for the paper because she honestly felt rehab would be better, even if attempted several times, than once in prison. She never dreamed she'd be thrust into prison herself. But when the story was written, she was still somewhat in denial about her own problem. Now she was straight, sober, clean, whatever the term is, and she still would be carted off to prison. It just wasn't fair.

Her mother and Ryan had come to visit her once she was in jail, but they didn't know what had happened earlier. That is, the bottle and counter incident. This would give her more time at Ohio Penitentiary for Women, she thought.

When she was ready to take her shower at the booking part of jail, she saw a bottle much like her old Tussionex bottles. The liquid was gold, it was on the counter from someone else's purse, and she eyed it with envy. She might need something to get her through the booking process and on to a solitary room it would be. So on her way to the shower, she looked around at the 20-some policemen and still did a very daring, stupid thing. She took her towel in her hand and snatched the bottle right under the noses of the personnel. There was a lady guard who escorted her into the shower who would leave her alone until she finished bathing, and she concealed the bottle under her towel until the guard left. Then before she began showering. She read the label and it was indeed Tussionex and the gold color shone through the container. It was about four ounces; had it been more, she probably couldn't have lifted it without someone noticing. But that small bottle . . . . Well, she saw it had about two ounces left, and she gulped it down in about three seconds. Unfortunately when she tried to hide it, the guard returned early.

"Are you finished with you shower . . . what's that in the corner?"

"What?"

"You liar, you junkie! I could be fired for this! You're going to get more time in OPW than you ever thought possible!"

Ridiculously, all Kym could think of was "my bad." She didn't say it, though. She just wished she'd hidden it better, although hiding places in the county shower were few and far between.

"When you are finished showering, I want you to go to medical. They will be sure you don't get any effects from what you've done. Hmmm, when this bottle was placed on the counter, there was about two ounces and now it's gone. you're in for a rude awakening, Mrs. Danzen. A REAL rude awakening."

Kym only hoped she could feel something from the dose before they did whatever they were going to do to her. When she was escorted to medical, two nurses and a doctor eyed her surreptitiously and told her what they were going to do.

"First, we are going to give you ipecac to make you puke your brains out. Then liquid charcoal to eliminate traces of the medicine from your body, If you are experiencing any good feelings you'll enjoy for about five minutes, because that's the maximum you will have to feel good about what you did—if you can. Now come into the examining room; we've got some ipecac to force down you."

Kym politely did as she was told. She drank the ipecac but only mild gagging occurred. The liquid charcoal—nicknamed charcoal tea—would finish the benefits of the cough syrup off

"If you don't drink the charcoal tea, we have ways to make you do so, including force-feeding."

Kym felt as if she were in Nazi Germany all of a sudden. She would cooperate, because she didn't want any other consequences, What a can of worms she opened. The charcoal tea was terrible, but a well-meaning nurse added a little bit of Coca Cola to it so it would be drinkable and not so nasty. They were right. In about ten minutes, the effects of any euphoria at all were gone, and now she was probably going to do 100 years in OPW.

CHAPTER ELEVEN

Kym had a slight sore throat from purging the ipecac, but in no way did she puke her brains out". She was led to a solitary cell upstairs on the second floor of the facility, and a sudden depression washed over her. She thought back when she had been in that horrific crash when she was 30. Some kids were drag racing and turned left of center into her Corvair (which has since been put out of production because there is no protection—more or otherwise—in the front. The Ford station nearly came into her front seat, and her face smashed against the dashboard. There were no seatbelt laws at the time, and if she had been wearing one, she probably would have not only destroyed her face, but her spleen as well. She remembered being in Akron Summit Hospital, and how she looked forward to the Demerol shots she received for her a torn-up face. She felt the same way as she did when she first took the Tussionex: optimistic, euphoric, happy, outgoing. She couldn't breathe out of her nose, but she still was doing okay until they changed the order to Darvon, and that just didn't feel the same.

So, she had been under the influence one other time before the cough syrup, she thought. She didn't know which was worse: being in the hospital or being in jail. People were more condescending and sympathetic when you're in the hospital, she thought. She wanted nothing more than a bottle of the syrup, but that was behind her now, probably forever.

She wondered, "Will my life ever be put back together just as my face was?" She sobbed softly and finally drifted off to sleep at lockdown time.

At 5 a.m., breakfast came. Everyone came out of their cells to wait in line, for shit on a shingle' (sausage gravy over a biscuit), a small helping of some kind of farina, milk, and orange juice. It wasn't too bad, but her appetite was just not there. Many of the girls were swearing like soldiers, laughing wildly, crying, yelling, or just about any other showdown behavior one could imagine, all except her. They asked her why she was so quiet and why didn't she want to speak to the others. Was she a snob? Was she better than they were? Her first thought was to answer, "From what I've seen and heard this morning, yes, I am," but her better judgment simply allowed her to reply.

"No, I'm just not feeling too well."

"Who is when we're here? You think you're different? Grow up!" came the reply from an obnoxious skinny girl of about 25. There seemed to be a clique among about ten inmates, and the others simply read and kept to themselves. A library was off to the side of the cells that contained battered or otherwise books in poor condition. Some missing pages. Still, she supposed it helped to pass the time in the Godforsaken state of being. Or was it just existing ? Around 10 a.m., a call came for Kym. She was to meet a public defender in the conference room.

She was led wearing handcuffs and a chain belt into the room and asked to sit down opposite a short gentleman with dark hair and a mustache. Somehow his spectacles made him seem smarmy.

Hello, Kym, I'm Atty. Barker. A public defender. I would like to speak with you about what happened to get you here."

"I was framed, sir. Plain and simple. If my urine was tested rightfully, it would have shown no alcohol and naltrexone would have appeared in the specimen. That didn't happen; therefore, it wasn't my specimen."

"But you cooked your goose when you took that bottle off the counter, Kym. That was theft. You originally were charged with deception to obtain a dangerous substance."

"I guess I thought that I was damned if I do use and damned if I don't. So I saw it, and took it, hoping for a little bit of euphoria before the depression set in as to everything that happened—that shouldn't have."

"Look, I don't know about a bad urine sample. That will have to be addressed at a later time, because nothing can be proven right now about a wrong or right specimen. But you never should have taken that bottle off the booking desk. That's going to cost you, plus they're still going to see you as an addict, regardless of whether you were—uh, framed or not. Everyone I have spoken to who knows about you here in booking wants to see you sent up the river for at least four years."

"Four years? Why did my use go against me, why did it make me a criminal? Now I wish everyone had taken my newspaper article to heart, because I'm a victim of something very wrong, and I'm the kind of person I wrote about. How ironic! I'd love to chuckle but frankly, I can't do that now."

"I'm going to lay it on the line, Kym. You will probably do four years in OPW, and I don't think you're going to get shock probation because of your little bottle theft and sticky fingers. The charge as deception', the second is theft. Even though it happened here in the booking room, it still constitutes stealing, and the fact it happened in view of 26 officers who screwed up by not paying attention to the evidence on their counter—whether it was yours or not—is not going to treat you kindly.

She indeed was screwed. No one would believe her about the frame-up now. She had to do something stupid that would affect her forever. And she knew the next trip to OPW was coming up in the morning.

"Attention, everyone come out of your cells to the sitting area!" boomed a loudspeaker at 5 p.m., just before the supper of dried up potatoes, fat-laden hamburger and kidney beans was served. When all were out in the area, the announcement came from the guard.

"The following inmates will be ready for transport to OPW at 4:30 tomorrow morning: Aster Smith, Jessica Traynor, Sylvia VanBuren, and Kymlin Corell. You will be given a trash bag to pack any needed objects in, although many of them will be replaced by the prison when you arrive."

She guessed that was the way to get rid of everybody's left-over junk—leave it to Summit Prison.

That night she dreamed about her youth, her childhood, and the dreams she had just a few short years ago. She wanted to be a Pulitzer winner, but now those newspaper days were long gone, as of 1990, when she announced her engagement to Ryan. Ryan, who had come to visit her in jail. What a surprise that was:—he'd found someone knew and was already sleeping with her. So much for ever getting together. The divorce was in the works, and his mother was springing for it. Can't dream about him anymore, and Barry is long gone—mentally, of course. She wasn't even attracted to the idea of ever seeing him again. She was a convicted felon now, and that would be with her forever, especially after the bottle theft of that little son of a gun that didn't even belong to her.

She finally fell asleep at 1:30 a.m., and remembered so many instances of growing up with her mother calling her "stupid" or "slow motion" or the like. Her self-esteem was never very high after those years, and she surmised that the lovely feeling the Tussionex gave her was a false or temporary fulfillment of a semblance of self-esteem.

She suddenly felt very alone. Her mother and Spencer had visited, but it was almost a token visit; they were ashamed of her, that much was evident. Ryan was out of the picture, of course. Even Atty. Gorner seemed to have disappeared after seeing the chambers sans Kym that day in Cooley's chambers. And the public defender had done nothing but told her how she'd blown it by stealing the infamous bottle. He wasn't about to help her. She had never gotten to see the judge, yet here she was, a couple hours before the OPW run. No one from Harvesters was there from day one, and why should they be? She had failed them, according to their lies. She truly was alone, except for the One she knew was there all the time God. She prayed that the trip and days afterward would not be too horrible, and that she would survive them.

Even though her family was not always the closest, Kym and Spence had been brought up in church, That meant so much to both of them, and they carried their faith throughout much of their life, although Kym seemed to have left Him at the front door whenever she pondered that lovely feeling from the syrup doses, Now she realized that He would see her through, no matter how horrible prison would be. It was God and Kym, together. Then the speaker sounded: "Time to get up and get moving those of you who are bound for OPW. Let's go!"

CHAPTER TWELVE

The four women were chained together with handcuffs and heavy chains reaching down past their knees, Their feet were bound with weights as well. There would be no escape for this non-fab four. Then they were led into a van, caged off from the driver's section so the females felt as if they were still behind bars. Kym felt so cheap, just as she had in her 12x12 ft. room at the jail.

She had a panic attack when the van left Akron, so certain her heart was going to give out—or break. Of course she was admonished for acting so dumb, both by the other women and the driver, and then she suddenly welled up with anger. She knew that Sylvia was going to OPW for life, because she had killed her husband in a bar with a nifty .38. The other two were drug dealers, mostly of the cocaine and LSD variety, with a little pot thrown in. Dear Jesus! Why was she going to prison? She asked herself over and over. She should have been more serious about the other four rehabs, she told herself, because her record had been lousy until she went to Harvesters. The one she finally determined would work for her sent her to OPW. Go figure. She even tried to pinch herself on the three-hour ride to Columbus just to wake up from this realistic dream, but as surreal as it was, it was really happening.

The driver teased the inmates by offering them something at McDonald's, and they eagerly ordered, thinking he really was having a heart. But he laughed in their faces as he gulped his Big Mac, mouth open to expose the half-chewed food, which almost made Kym ill. He told them they would be dining in the ever-luxurious OPW cafeteria, and also would be working there for long hours, It seemed every inmate was broken in' by carrying heavy trays of food, sweeping and mopping the entire cafeteria (often with straight bleach, which was a great way to sting your eyes), serving hundreds of other inmates, then cleaning and mopping all over again. This was the job most hated by inmates, because it was much more tiring than any other, especially after cleaning the gym-sized food room.

Kym as ironically transported to OPW on her birthday, October 16, 1996, and the only compensation for the endless ride was observing the gorgeous trees heavy with fall colors. Tears in her eyes, she thanked God for the panorama in a whisper. She knew that there was still beauty in the world, which seemed almost nil these days. But she hadn't seen nothing' yet. And this does not refer to beauty.

The van pulled up alongside the barbed, curved-in-circles endless fence, where the guard station was placed. A stout, balding guard in a gray uniform beckoned the driver through the gate, where he drove to a building among many on the compound. This was the check-in place, where mug shots were taken and showers were offered, or rather, mandatory, but there was no time to enjoy them.

They were timed at three minutes each, including shampooing, Shirts were given to the women: green for minimum status, which Kym wore, pink for medium blue for maximum or orange for ultra max. Sylvia woe the orange shirt. There was nothing fancy about the get-up. Each woman was issued state-made khaki pants (three pair) and 3 shirts, plus three underwear panties and a couple of ill-fitting bras. Socks and shoes were given as well. Nothing was as drab as those outfits, because after all, no one special graced OPW.

The next stop was the Admissions Building across the campus. Kimlyn was fine with the clothes, but it took her aback when she was fingerprinted like a common criminal—which she guessed she now was. Anyway, she was eager to settle into whatever room she would have. Hopefully it would be a single cell like the other one, or perhaps a double, which wouldn't be too awful. She was told she would only be in Admissions for about two weeks, then on to a permanent" place called a cottage" where she would be a part of population. One building at a time. When she saw what her digs would be at Admissions, she almost puked. There was row after row of beds, about 59 per row and just behind those were fifty more. People were packed like sardines, and the building had a couple of fans to keep the huge room cool. But there was a not one iota of privacy. Altogether, the rows constituted about 300 inmates, and the only area that could be called one's own was a small single bed, half of a bunk bed. Each woman was issued a lock box for her belongings, mostly those issued at the clothing area, were kept. These were personals like toothbrushes, combs, and other things considered necessities. The rest were to be bought using the inmates' own funds at the commissary building, so the first month's pay of about $20 would go for razors, lotions, shampoo, makeup of those who thought it necessary, hairbrushes, toothpaste, coffee, and other everyday articles. So the only area on the floor that was considered each person's own was her lockbox, kept under the bed, and her bed area, which must be made perfectly every morning. Soon jobs would be issued, but for the first few days everyone was a "porter" or housekeeper. If even a penny was found on anyone's person, that would mean a trip to the "hole", a very dismal two-person room with very few privileges and noted for fights when one of the dwellers had too much of the other roommate. Kym was to find out much more as her acquaintance with OPW was made and familiarity bred contempt.

CHAPTER THIRTEEN

Kym wondered how anyone could sleep in this place. Between the snoring, coughing, yelling, screaming, laughing, and noise of constant lockbox opening, she thought sleep would never come. She did her assigned porter job and went to the cafeteria for dinner once she was settled. Johnny Marzettii, peaches and corn were served, with Kool Aid for the beverage, She didn't realize just how tired she was becoming. She went into the restroom where about five toilets served 1800 inmates (with some four sinks), and undressed in one of the stalls. A shapeless sheet with two arm holes served as a nightgown, so everyone went around looking like ghosts. They were not to go in the recreation room unless fully dressed, but she didn't feel like playing cards (she really didn't know much about card games anyway), Scrabble, or just talking to some of the women who bragged about how they got here.

Everyone had to be in their beds at 9:30 for countdown, then could go back into the rec room if they desired, but she had already gotten in her "ghost gown" and wanted to try to get some sleep. The bright fluorescents stayed on all the time until about midnight, when it was lights out. Fortunately Kym was on the bottom bunk, which shielded her from the brightest, most direct lighting, and she actually fell asleep almost immediately, as tired as she was. Tomorrow will take care of itself, as the Bible said, she thought.

Just as in jail, 5:00 a.m. was wake-up time, if breakfast was desired. With so many people using the bathroom, getting ready seemed very slow, but finally things would come together. The showers had to be completed in three minutes, as they did upon arrival at the facility. There were no showers at any other time except right after dinner or before breakfast when the line was timed in the showers. That included getting dry and dressed in the stalls. Kym never felt clean. Today's menu would be as always. boiled eggs, toast, cereal and juice or milk. That was the most normal meal of the day. After returning from the quarter-mile walk to and from the cafeteria, it was porter's time to mop and wash floors, walls, inmate quarters and the like. Also of course, she had to scrub toilets, but thankfully not with a toothbrush. At least they had a heart on this matter, But she dreaded the time when this could change into a full-fledged army barracks.

Lunch was soup and sandwiches, with gingerbread. It sounded better than it was. After dinner—spaghetti and meatballs, minimal tomato sauce, garlic bread and cheese—she was ready to read a book she found in the Admissions library with only about twenty pages missing. She would just have to guess how Brindle's Lover turned out to be.

She saw one or two girls she had seen back at Summit Jail, but she had nothing in common with the slang and jargon they used, so she just smiled and would say hello, If anyone tended to become an introvert, this would be the place to foster it, providing you were a smart person.

Before trying to sleep, she reminisced among the noise with all her senses about her childhood and he life she lived as a pre-teen. She grew up in East Akron, and would ride her SMF Roadmaster bicycle up to Snappy Hamburgs every other day to obtain those old fashioned, tiny hamburgers for her folks, Spence, and herself. She could almost smell the French fries and salt, taste the rich chocolate shake that was hand-made, and sniff the grease that made for cholesterol-filled but delicious little meat patties with mustard and onions. She felt the gravel beneath her feet as she drove her bike onto the sidewalk from the driveway and up the sidewalk to the little restaurant carry-out. Most of the houses were still in that area, which never seemed to change. It was at 13 that her father had been promoted to a vice president of First Second Bank, as well as being a district manager of its operations, and they had moved to the west side, Kym liked both areas, but the west side offered a better school system. She was in National Honor Society, honor roll, and other organizations while in Canterbury High School, and she loved studying. At that time, :The Man From U.N.C.L.E. was on TV, and she adopted the persona of Illya Kuryakin, bookworm and introvert extraordinaire. Later in college she knew what it was to be outgoing, and from her freshman year in college until graduation she became the life of the party and liked it. She was in a singing group and choir at church, and enjoyed graduation year as a student teacher for sixth grade. She had a lot of friends then, and now she was among 300 women and very lonely. What a contrast.

Each day seemed pretty much the same Cinderella style bullied cleaning routine, but now she was told to report to the cafeteria at 5 a.m. to begin working.

Everything she heard about the cafeteria was true. The bleach to clean floors that was not watered down and took away your breath, the cockroaches, unclean conditions, lugging heavy food containers back and forth serving hundreds of a matter of minutes and cleaning everything all over again.

She endured this job for about five weeks, and then something happened one day in early summer of '96. She had been placed in population with another 300 women who shared her quarters, so no privacy was to exist, and the cafeteria was seemingly surreal in some weird way that day.

"What is happening to me? I feel as though blinders or curtains are coming down over my eyes and a bunch of gnats are circling me. What are those black specks? I don't understand what's happening to my eyes. I've got to talk to a CO."

Her cafeteria shift was nearly over, so she waited until she could get back to her cottage, then went to the Corrections Officer known as Miss Andrews.

"Ma'am something is wrong with my eyes, and I really need to get them checked. Please, can you help me? I need to see Dr. Mackey as soon as possible. I might be going blind."

"Let me check you records . . . . here they are. you're due in a month for an eye exam. No, you cannot go any sooner. If I did that for you, I'd have to do it for everyone. You probably just need some sleep."

Her heart sank. What was going to happen to her? She did not need more rest. She had been getting enough sleep after she told herself her nightly snoring was no worse than her father's had been. Others had complained about Elvie's snoring, and the complaints had been the only thing that had awakened her. She simply was not lacking rest; she was going blind and there was no one to talk with who would understand.

Somehow she got through the next month, counting the days until her appointment. Today was finally the day, and she praised God that the day was finally here. She walked over to medical.

After being called into his office, Dr. Mackey gave her a brief exam, then leaned back with a very concerned look on his face. His opinion?

"You have a detached retina. Why didn't you come over sooner? We're going to try to save as much of your sight as possible, but you must realize that since you waited a month, you'll probably lose some eyesight. We're going to have you on transport this afternoon for Columbus Center for Hospital Inmates. Hurry and go pack, you'll be there several days."

She was both overjoyed that something was finally to be done about her dilemma and furious that she might lose sight because a stupid CO was so apathetic about her appointment. But now she was ready to go.

She packed a few toiletries and reported for transport. In a couple of hours she was ready for surgery, settled into the small but efficient inmate medical building. When she returned, she would have it out with Miss Andrews, even though it probably meant a trip to the hole.

Of course nothing would be done about Miss Andrews. She was just the right combination of apathetic and smart-ass to make it as a CO. Kymlin was in surgery at 3:48 that afternoon. She should have been there 28 days earlier. Apparently inmates were less than human to the guard population.

She emerged with a multitude of bandages over her right eye. She joked with the doctor that she was one of those Arrrh Matey kind of pirates. He did not smile. She lost her smile petty quickly, and realized that the eye hurt a bit severely, She was transported back to her room, whom she shared with a very nice older lady named Corrinna, for whom she was very grateful. They kept each other company after Corrinna had her gallbladder out. At least Kym didn't have to have something like that done, too.

Codeine was given to her the week she was in the hospital, and she was grateful for the small buzz it provided, even though it wasn't Tussionex. Her eye became much better, and the day finally came when she was transported back to OPW. The estimate was that she'd lost about 25 per cent of her sight in the right eye, but her left one was still very strong with lenses. Had she been able to have surgery within 48 hours of the floaters and blinders effect, she would have lost very little, perhaps two per cent at most. If she were a pugilist, Miss Andrews could look forward to a decking, but she was not a fighter and shuddered to think that someday she might have to turn into one. She had a weird feeling that the day was coming, but she had no inkling of when or where. Oh, well.

The day after transport back to OPW and Hazel Cottage was one of the most trying evenings of her life. The cottage was located in a basement setting, and the rain began. The sidewalk leading to Hazel were being bombarded with water, and the water was running down the steps like Niagara Falls, Petty soon the cottage was becoming flooded with rain up to six inches deep as it kept creeping in. Women were stationed to use brooms and brush it back outside, but this was to no avail. Lockboxes were placed on top of beds, and mattresses were ready for passage to the gymnasium. How would they be transported? The inmates would carry them, plus their lockboxes. It was a good thing the mattresses wee only about three inches thickly Kym and her neighbors lifted their mattresses over their shoulders, carrying their lockboxes in their other hands. God help those who had bought much commissary supplies last week. Some of the lockboxes had already been infiltrated with water, and some of the women's only belongings were completely soaked and dripping, Some of the ladies were lucky enough to find a laundry bin in which the lockboxes could be placed while the mattresses stayed over one shoulder, but this was he exception and not the rule Kym was praying her eye surgery would not come undone with the heavy double load she was wielding, but they had to vacate the building fast or the water would have been deep enough to swim in, While the girls threw their mattresses, blankets, and lockboxes down together, on the hard gym floor, they noticed the gymnasium was also leaking. Water was coming down the walls. Fortunately, it didn't come into the gym as far as the middle of the floor, and though the floor was hard, it was dry. The harsh lights stayed on all night, and when daylight came, it was time to go back to Hazel. They don't know how it was accomplished, but the dry van clan brought in their machines and actually cleaned most of the water from the building. The big problem left to the girls was MUD, and the whole floor was s complete mud puddle. Everyone placed their mattresses on the bedsprings and grabbed mops and brooms to rid the old cottage of the mud all around their feet in their living quarters. It wasn't easy. This was considered just a medium-class emergency; things could become much worse, and would. Thank heavens it wouldn't be in Kym's cottage.

She praised God for sparing her eyesight during the exodus to and fro the gym, and asked that the crisis not happen again. Sometimes the women were stationed with their brooms and mops to chase the water out, but at least they never had to carry all their belongings like the Jews out of Egypt.

The next crisis came following a letter from Atty. Gorner stating that because Kym had stolen that bottle of Tussionex from the counter while in booking, she would be denied shock probation, and would have to do all four years in OPW. She had written to everyone including the governor about the frame-up, but no one dared tackle Judge Cooney. When she thought about it more, she realized what the problem was: Judge Cooney had begun the Class AA farm baseball team that would feed into the Cleveland Indians, and because of her great contribution to the sports world, no one wished to pursue dogging her.

That was not the crisis, however, After eating chicken in the cafeteria one afternoon, Kym heard a server on that shift say that the chicken was bad and should be thrown out. Of course, that came after her friends and she had eaten it. No one died, but several inmates had a nasty bout of salmonella for several weeks. Still, she had to work, work, work. She lost track of the number of restroom trips, and lost about twenty pounds over the next month.

She had been miserable that month. She wondered if Lady Luck would ever smile on her. Then she heard of some inmates worse off than she was, and her countenance was humble but grateful it wasn't her more things had happened to.

Her cottage was not far from the Lifers building, and she knew that four years was not an eternity, that she could bear it if she absolutely had to. She had heard horror stories that turned out to be true because they were verified by the guards who remembered them. For instance, one girl was pregnant by a CO and tried to abort the baby with a coat hanger. She later died of infection. Another inmate had hanged herself. Kym wondered how the lifers took prison life day after day after day,

Through all this, she yearned for something to make her feel better. She actually ate bark off trees and chewed up flowers to see if they held any euphoric qualities. She made an excuse to go back over to the B building where she was helping write an OPW newsletter, but it was not the newsletter she was interested in on that particular day.

There were lots of morning glories along the pathway, and she heard the seeds were similar to LSD, so she gathered several seeds and brought them back to Hazel with her. Having endured bouts of diverticulosis for several yes, all the seeds did was make her almost as sick as when she had salmonella. Others had seen her do this, and began reporting the incident to the Hazel COs, The last straw came when she tried to barter her commissary for some cough syrup from a medium rank inmate who said the "shit was really good stuff.". Unfortunately, the cough syrup was plain old Robitussin, because anything stronger was not issued at OPW, and this incident was witnessed, too,

At about the same time, Kym refused to work again in the cafeteria because she blamed all the heavy lifting and bleach for her detached retina. She soon had a chance to view the "hole" from the inside.

"What have I done? I feel so stupid, and now everyone will think I'm some sort of nutcase," she reckoned to herself. She was led with handcuffs and escorted by a CO to the worst portion of the hole where there was one room below ground level that was no warmer than 50 degrees. She was on her period, too, and had no change of clothes or underwear to help her get through those few days. She developed bronchitis and was actually afraid she was going to die. A kindly CO brought her some extra blankets, but they were not enough to stave off the cold, dank atmosphere of that tiny little room,

While she was there, two maximum security inmates were brought in for fighting, and they were sent to the more bearable open room upstairs. Kym inquired as to why she was not sent there as a minimum security, and the reply was that the guards :had to keep an eye on the two mischief makers. So they were getting a better room because they were fighting. It made no sense.

CHAPTER FOURTEEN

Kym received some mail, but the little cold room was so dark she couldn't even read it. Even the tiny sink had nothing but cold water. Just when she was resigned to dying of pneumonia, she was whisked off to a two-person room and had a bearable roommate. But she really did fear that her bronchitis was breaking into pneumonia.

"This must be the room the two troublemakers left," she thought sarcastically. It was better than the one she'd had, certainly, because at least there was a bed rather than just a cold mattress, a sink, and toilet which were standard size, One of the COs told Kym that the room she spent three days in was condemned and was going to be destroyed, Great news after she moved,

Once she was in the better room, she realized that she could not buy commissary or that she had none of the privileges that she had in population. One girl who apparently was there for life would sing "The Rose" over and over again, She had a beautiful voice, but after the first 25 times you'd like to hear something different, said Kym to her bunkmate Rosie, a rather backward but nice girl. Rosie was in the hole for getting jealous over her lady love and threatening to kill her. Kym knew this girl was not capable of carrying out any such threats, but just saying something about killing was enough to launch her into the hole.

For the two weeks she was there, Kym found Rosie to be pleasant, and whenever the book cart rolled around with even more decrepit books than were available in the regular OPW library, they both eagerly took several to pass the time,

A shower was offered in a tiny booth in front of everyone (although a curtain was pulled across the booth), and three minutes was again the time OPW thought it took to get a good shower. At least they were offered every day,

Meals were brought to the cells; there was no fellowshipping except for the bunkmate each person had. Except for the showers, inmates stayed in their rooms 24/7. Many exercised to pass the time.

Kym found out her bunkie had smuggled some nerve pills (tranquilizers) inside the cell in a tiny bit of plastic in her he vagina, and both girls were tempted to take them when they went stir crazy, The thought of the pills being in that area of Rosie's body turned Kym off, but she overcame her gagging reflex and took one of the pills. It made her feel very relaxed. Rosie let her have one more, but that was all.

Kym had a conversation with Rosie later that day about a subject she had never gotten into: homosexuality. Rosie approached her with, "You know, it's really lonely here. There are 1900 women which is twice as many as at this place is supposed to hold, but ya know what? It's twice as many to choose from." Choose from? For what?

"Having a woman, silly! A girlfriend. Lots of inmates substitute women for men because the pickings are all around us, and there are all kinds of women here. Some are pretty hot. What do you think, Kym?"

"Well, I had a guy back home but he divorced me. I'm still not attracted to women though."

"Why don't you give it a try? I, for one, am willing to have a relationship. And please don't take me wrong, Kym, but you aren't a bad looking lady. Your blonde hair, shoulder length, is to die for. And your smile is genuine, not pasted on. You are quite attractive. Would you consider it in the near future? Perhaps when we get out of here and back to population?"

"I . . . I don't think so, but I'm very uh . . . honored that you said such nice things about me."

"Yeah, well, that's the way it goes. You know, some women almost force others to be their better half. I've seen strong women jerk around—and I mean physically—their girlfriends. There isn't love there, just someone to take away some of the lonely hours. But it's better than stagnating and keeping to yourself all the time." Kym knew this last statement was directed toward her, because she had become quite the loner of her cottage. She just didn't want to say or do something that could be misconstrued or taken offensively.

"Are you straight or gay, Rosie? And am I really attractive in your eyes? It somehow fascinates me."

"I'm straight, but now I guess I've had some female crushes. I'd never threaten them or warn them to stay away from anyone else, though. That happens. People here get petty possessive. Sometimes it's all they can hang onto."

"How does this thing work? With all the guards watching, is there any time to be intimate?"

"Mostly the stalls. If you walk in and see four feet instead of two, you won't be viewing a congenital set of conjoined twins."

The stalls are so small. How . . . "

Rosie cut her off.

"Look, Kym, I don't really know what happens in thee. But the showers—now that's another story."

"Is that when the real heavy stuff happens?"

"Oh, yeah. That's mostly oral and finger-poke junk, but it turns you on."

Kym suddenly felt strange, not because she didn't want to understand the gay relationship, but because she was trying to understand privacy in a shower stall that wouldn't send someone to the hole. They had to be mighty careful—and quick.

"I think I'll just keep things light, Rosie. Rely on myself. I've never experimented before."

"Oh. All right then."

What if Rosie had a sudden mean steak and forced Kym to do something she didn't want to? Sort of a split-personality bi-polar thing. Rosie's eyes looked tired, and Kym took that to mean she was just another woman trying to get along at OPW, which she was.

Kim thanked God that she was not some sort of wrestler type who could force her down on the bunk with something else in mind. She'd heard the horror stories of other cottages' inmates, but then again, she'd also seen couples who seemed very content, so it all depended which was the luck of the draw. But for Kym, she kept herself company.

A few days later, a verbal incident occurred that really humiliated Kym. She had polycystic ovaries and this caused hair follicles to appear in places usually found on a man, especially the chin and face. After being in the hole for a week, her hair had started to be noticeable. One male CO came to the door with offers of a shower at that time. He looked at Kym and burst out laughing. Oh, yeah—you're the one with the beard! Have you been sleeping that much in your cell to get it that long, Rip Van Winkle?"

She was angry, but didn't cry. She was offered a razor to use under close scrutiny of a female CO, which she did. But in a few days it would be back; of course, she might be out of the hole and back with her own beloved razor at Hazel Cottage by then, she hoped.

CHAPTER FIFTEEN

After doing a month in the hole (including that below-ground room known as the pit"), she was released.

The days came and went, but didn't exactly speed by. She was surprised to note that on a calendar by the end of April, she would have been at OPW two easy, or half the time she was sentenced to spend at OPW.

After vowing she would never work in the cafeteria again because of her eye that was most likely caused by all the heavy lifting, Kym was sent to the hole three more times, all because she was trying to protect her eyes. Finally, after being told she had really bucked the protocol worse than anyone ever had before, she won her vow to become a G.E.D. tutor, and truly enjoyed putting on newspaper seminars, having the women write stories (some were quite poignant), and teaching them grammar. This was truly the high point of prison, because she was helping others to make something of themselves. But she never understood why she had to buck the cafeteria so much before they finally placed her in the tutorial job! She thought they just wanted to control their inmates, but finally she had given them run for their money and began to teach. She loved doing what she could for the students.

Unfortunately the tutorial program came to an end, none of the inmates knew why. Apparently money for funding the program was at a minimum, so all the tutors either went back to work in the cafeteria, or as porters (which Kym was ordered to be).

"Hmph, the first great thing about this dismal place and it's kicked right in the head. If this is a penitentiary (meaning penitence-teaching), it had a long way to go."

Day after day, Kym did her porter job, cleaning, mopping, dusting, emptying trash, the whole routine. Then one morning her stomach began to hurt so much she almost doubled over with pain. She was told to finish her jobs before she could rest. She hurried along, then went back to her bunk. She was prepared to run to the restroom in case she threw up, but so far the pain did not indicate puking.

She wasn't able to eat lunch or dinner, and by evening the pain had her doubled over, in the fetal position on her bunk.

"Oh, dear God, please help me," she screamed, upsetting many of the other inmates. A call went down to the inmate hospital she had been in for her eye over in Columbus. She was to be on transported at 6 a.m. tomorrow morning. There were, fortunately, other inmate patients who had gastrointestinal upsets and that was a major reason for this trip. In other words, her condition fit right in.

She grimaced, cried, and nearly screamed all the way on the 40-mile trip. She was grateful she didn't have to wait a month now as she did when she lost part of her eyesight. She supposed being noisy had something to do with the hurried trip. Most people don't want to listen to a sobbing or yelling from an inmate suffering from abdominal cramps.

When everyone disembarked from the prison bus, they were led to a large waiting room. They had to wait at least an hour, before the earlier group as finished.

Then, with handcuffs and chains, she was called to be seen. The guard unlocked the connecting chains from her that grouped the four women together. She was led to a small examining room, where x-rays were taken. And taken, they were. There must have been 12 of her abdomen and stomach. Why so many?" she asked after the initial exam.

"I suspect your gallbladder is acting up. It may have to come out," the doctor said. "The x-rays and cat scan you just had taken show some considerable damage and stones. That baby will have to come out. But we don't do gallbladders here. You'll have to go to a regular' hospital later today, we'll make arrangements with Columbus State Medical Facility for you. You will be transported in about an hour."

"I've never had gallbladder trouble before," Kymlin said Are you sure that's what it is?"

"Yes, quite certain. We can send the copies of x-rays and cat scan along with you, where your guard can keep track of it. Don't worry. You'll be fine. There are considerable stones, too, so I think a larger hospital with specific abdominal and gastrointestinal offices and exam rooms will be the best. They can operate and have you on your way the next day"

Her green eyes winced with pain as she was transported, and she was immediately taken to the abdominal area. She had heard talk about gallbladders bursting and was alarmed.

The hospital had a special floor for inmates, because after all, they had on orange jumpsuits, handcuffs, and looked as if they were going to rob a bank. "Normal" patients didn't want to see that. The care would be good, at least Kym certainly hoped so, as they prepped her on a gurney before taking her to the O. R. She was going to be placed in a bed had recently used by a girl with tuberculosis, and Kym hoped they had scrubbed the bed down thoroughly. It was hard to pinpoint, but the care, although adequate, was different than what she'd seen on the way up to the sixth "inmate" floor. A caste system was evident in America, don't let anyone fool you. We were just numbers, numbers who were probably guinea pigs upon whom operations were done by resident surgeons. Interesting. Hope they had been here quite some time. They seemed apathetic, but chances are, they were just businesslike and serious. She knew no one would practice at such a fine hospital if they were below average. But she chuckled to herself just before surgery, even with all the pain, thinking of a sign on the sixth floor right after exiting an elevator: SIXTH FLOOR: INMATES TO PRACTICE ON, FEEL FREE."

Of course the sign was in her head, but to make her chuckle with the terrific pain she was enduring, the thought had to be pretty amusing. To her it was.

CHAPTER SIXTEEN

Kym awoke with some pain, but not as much as she anticipated after losing her gallbladder. She was told that the quality of her food lately was so full of cholesterol that if her gallbladder had never presented problems, now was the time. So not only was her eye problem the result of prison, so was her gallbladder.

The next day Kym was expected to walk right out of the hospital and into the waiting prison van, which was at least a walk of one-third mile, from bed to parking lot to van. But the pain was now very dull, and she had been given no pain killers. Soon it would be back to portering at Hazel Cottage for the next several months. But she looked at a calendar, and realized she only had one more year to go until release date. The time was creeping, but it was advancing, even if very very slowly,

Karaoke was something Kym enjoyed, and one of the few activities that was right up her alley. She loved to sing to all the ladies, "Harper Valley P.T.A.", the Jeannie C. Riley song of the early '70s. She could belt it out with the best of them—and some of the singers weren't bad. Before she left in May '98, she established herself as the "Harper Valley singer", and that tickled her for a while. Hmmm, I DID do a pretty good job of it, didn't she? Ha ha!"

Monday morning she was in a bad mood because one woman had snored all night and, being a light sleeper, she couldn't get to sleep for more than twenty minutes at a time. She headed for breakfast, and the women from her cottage all got in line. Just when it was almost time for the green shirts to be served, a barrage of maximum security women cut right in front of them. Kym was in no mood for this breach of etiquette or just plain manners, so she told the lead woman to go to the back of the line with her cronies. She couldn't stand this person, and most others couldn't either. A very pretty but tough blonde, Glinda was a lifer who grew jealous of her husband's continued attention toward her baby son. Because she couldn't stand the family competition, Glinda took her baby, Harry, and nuked him to death in the microwave. When her husband asked what was for dinner, Glinda hissed, "Your son—you're eating him!"

Just as Kym told her to get back in line, she shoved Kym against the wall and laughed. That was all she could take from this bitch. She came back into the line and decked Glinda while everyone cheered and began calling her "Rambo" (which she disdained). The rest of the maxes went to the back of the line, and Kym yelled to them "Anyone else?" with her fists clenched. No one challenged her. And that was the end of the great Glinda encounter of the breakfast line.

The next few months went a bit faster, and Kym began to count the days until she would be released on May 5, 1998. There were loads of incidents that really didn't mean the end of the world, as when one inmate of Hazel had lice and everyone in the place had to take showers and shampoo right away, three minutes per person, of course. No one else caught them—at least, not that day.

The months passed and finally she was one day away from leaving. She had made friends with a young girl of 23 named Sophia, who invited her to come up to Ashtabula when she was released. Sophia as released in March, and went back to live with her mother and son. Kym decided she did not want to return to Akron, but try something different in a new place where she could help teach Sophia how to read and to get over the stigma of being mentally challenged. She had tutored her often in OPW, and the invitation was extended for Kym's release in May. She could be on her own, begin in a new area, and help Sophia in exchange for rent. She was also to get food stamps which she could share as well.

She bade goodbye to those she had tutored and the few women who meant friendship to her, and was taken to Cleveland to catch the Ashtabula bus. She carried a trash bag full of the things she wanted to keep, but there were very few she considered valuable indeed. She truly was starting on her own in a town she knew nothing about.

CHAPTER SEVENTEEN

When she found herself in the Rent A Center that served as a tiny bus terminal in Ashtabula, she only had to wait about fifteen minutes, and then she saw Sophia and her significant other pull in the parking lot. They bid hello, then they took her home. What she didn't know was that Denny lived with them in a very small apartment, and that Sophia was pregnant now. She knew that Denny had a high-paying trucker job, but with Sophia and her mother Estelle receiving welfare (Medicaid), she suspected he was living there illegally. Oh, well, there were more important things to worry about.

Sophia had made the apartment sound very apropos, but it was indeed small and she found she would be sleeping on the living room couch. The youngster she was also to tutor, Sophia's six-year-old son, was deeply disturbed, going around in the apartment threatening to kill everybody, including Kym. His grades were atrocious, and she didn't know how she would start training this little devil.

Sophia asked her about her assets.

'Kym, did your mother send your food stamps yet? You can share them with us as your rent when they come," I thought tutoring was going to pay my rent."

"Well, that will help, but you said when you arrived here your mother would help out. We're not rich, Kym. You're gonna have to help us,"

Kym was becoming a little disillusioned. She thought she might as well share the stamps because she would be eating some of the food, so she reasoned she could do it. It was fairly late when she was picked up at the terminal, and she was tired so she lay down on the couch early. Everyone was noisy, playing the radio, TV, swearing up a storm, and virtually ignoring her. The next day she was pressed to look for a job, which she wanted to do anyway, but the pressure from Sophie and her family was nothing short of tacky and disrespectful,

Ah, but there was one thing Sophie had promised Kym when she came to stay: cough syrup, They both knew the value of Tussionex, but Kym would have to make an appointment with Sophie's doctor if she wanted any. Lucky she was armed with about $100 she'd saved from her tutoring and porter jobs.

She had given Sophie's address to her mom, and Sophie's mom was still pressuring Kym for food stamps Kym's mom had saved. The food stamps belonged to Spencer, who was out of work, but he had given them to their mother so she could buy what she needed. With her father gone, things were not easy.

On the third day the stamps were in Kym's hands—and observed by Sophie and Estelle. They began to badger her once again.

Kym, how much did she send? We all have to eat, and you know we don't make anything with no one working. Can you . . . "

Hold it a minute! What about Denny? doesn't he work for the trucking place?"

Uh, sometimes. But he won't get paid for about a month. We really need whatever stamps you have that you can share. In fact, there is a little grocery store next door called The Shopping Gig". Will you go over and bring us some food? You know what I like, and Mom will eat the same, Dusty will share. Can you do this now? We don't have very much right now."

Kim had started to feel she had come to live with a bunch of leeches, but she complied because there was no place else to go. She bought some cereal, milk, juice, mat, bread, and fruit. She knew this was a pretty balanced group of groceries.

They had all gone someplace when she came in the door, so she unpacked the foods and waited to show what she had bought with them. They couldn't find fault with THIS stuff. So she relaxed and waited until they came home from whatever excursion they had been on.

Dusty opened the cabinets. What did you get? Where's the good stuff? What's wrong with you? I'll bet you didn't even buy ice cream!"

When Sophie and Estelle perused the supply, they, too, seemed disappointed. They said everything was just okay, but they knew she had some money too and why didn't she buy some booze?

"I didn't know any of you drink. Look—there's all kinds of wholesome stuff here. it's . . . "

A waste! Couldn't you do any better than this? No one is going to eat this stuff. Where's the French fries, TV dinners, easy stuff? Ph, well, guess you didn't know. We can eat this, so don't worry this time. But now you know."

"Sophie, I made an appointment with Dr. Hastings for tomorrow afternoon. Can you take me? You said if I made it for Thursday that you could take me, if it was afternoon."

"Can't. But there are buses that go by our house all the time. You can catch one at three and be at the doctor's by four. It IS Dr. Hastings, right? he'll give you something, don't worry!"

Kym felt her money was going to go down in record time, but the bus was only fifty cents. She was relieved to see the office, never having been there before It seemed every time the going got tough, Kym got going—to doctors. And this was so many years later. She did her little bronchitis cough trick. She also told Dr. Hastings that she was a friend of the Steelmen's, so he would know she just didn't come from out of the blue. The first time she saw Dr. Hastings, he prescribed Hycodan, a similar syrup to the liquid gold. But not quite as strong. Still, she had eight ounces to help he through the new nightmare that may be forming at Sophia's house for her. She couldn't understand why she still craved this medicine so much, considering what it had done to her and where it had led her. But the fascination with the "feeling" was still there, especially when days seemed to be rather unpleasant. Her two landladies decided to bug her at every turn, to try and get money from her. They were relentless about her finding a job. (After all, Danny was the only one working in the household, and that was illegal as far as insurance would be concerned); she needed to pay rent now, because she found out the boy was impossible to teach, He was greatly disturbed, and would stand on Sophia's car while screaming at Kym, I'm gonna kill you!"

One night he would not leave her alarm clock alone, so Kym threatened him with a smack to the derriere if he persisted, When Sophia found out, she told Kym, "No ONE threatens my son." Guess that's why he was such a nasty little brat, thought Kym.

After searching and treading the streets every day from 9 until 6, Kim had some prospects of jobs but none definite as yet. She was harassed by the two selfish women and their awful boy until worse came to worst. Kym watched the females smoke pot, sell drugs out of the home, and when Danny came home, he and Sophie would smoke crack, oblivious to anyone else around. Had it not been for one incident, Kym would have been long gone. This is what happened.

Sophia had some pregnancy complications and was placed in the hospital. Kym went along to encourage her, but Sophia was hysterical.

"Why are you so worried? Your pregnancy is going along well; this is just a small glitch in the time," Kym inquired.

Apparently Sophie had estimated wrong, and her baby was almost due now rather than in a month.

"You don't understand, Kym! I've been on pot and if they find that in my tests they will seek foster care for my baby! You've got to help me, and there's one way to do it."

Estelle urged Kym to substitute her urine sample for Sophie's, since they were not looking for cough syrup but illegal drugs.

"Aw, c'mon, Sophie! I can't do that with a clear conscience!"

"If you want to stay in our home for another day you'd better cooperate," hissed Estelle.

Kym had no choice. She had been job searching but not house hunting and she would be homeless if she were forced out of her temporary home.

"All right, but this does not set well with me. Give me the urinal."

Of course the urine tested negative for pot, and everyone was happy but they didn't say anything to Kym. They acted as if she was simply expected to do it, that they were indulging her with a house for now. She was forbidden to tutor Larry by Estelle and Sophie. She couldn't take much more of this crap.

The baby came in two weeks. Her name was Dixie Lynn. Everyone fawned and smiled at her with no thought of Kym's doing what she did to save Dixie's hide from going into a foster home. Or to save Sophie's and Estelle from possible prison. Every time Kym wanted to hold little Dixie, the answer was no. She was being passed from Estelle to Sophie to Danny to Larry, but Sophie was jealous Kym would bond with her before Sophie did.

"They wouldn't even have this child if it weren't for that stunt I had to do," she thought with vehemence, for a change. She was beginning to dislike the Steelman family and their friends. But she still did not have a job. Not yet.

One day it all came crashing down around her. She told the women she was sick and tired of all the drugs being passed, and all of them were going to go to jail if this didn't cease.

"Why? Are you gonna tell the police?" chortled Estelle.

"I think she's serious, Ma. She may have told them already."

"Look, I haven't told anyone, but your habits are gonna come back to haunt you, and they'll see that I am using just what put me in prison, and, well, it just has to stop,"

"I think she HAS told, Ma. I'm going to get the gun in the bedroom," Estelle said nothing else until she began to chant Bitch, Bitch, Bitch . . . " and Sophie came out with a .38 in her hand.

"Oh, no! I haven't told anyone, I was trying to tell you are in danger with all this trafficking . . . . " Suddenly Sophie was like a madwoman. She raced at Kym, who fortunately was near the bathroom. Kym ran into the bathroom just as the door slammed and the door handle flew off,

"I'm dead, dead, now I'm out of prison and I'm dead, what do I do, what do I do . . . "

Just then, she heard Sophie retreat. She didn't know what that meant, but she decided to come out of the bathroom and try to reason with these crazies, If possible. The next thing she knew, Sophie was gathering all her clothes that had been given her by a thrift shop to search for a job, and threw them onto the yard. She quickly tossed everything that was Kym's outside, Kim was dumbfounded at all this behavior, but she knew something would happen one of these days. It finally had. The two females stared at her and told her to get out: one chubby, bleached blond, heavyset, raging blue eyes and wearing a muumuu; the other tall, thin, dark brown hair and somewhat of a left-over tummy bulge from the pregnancy with Dixie. Hard to believe the blonde was Sophie's mom, She was dressed like a hooker, and so was Sophie. It was all so atrocious.

Finally, Kym found herself homeless. Just she was ready to walk, her friend Robin from job searching drove by. They picked up all her outside clothes and placed them in a trash bag supplied by Sophie, who had calmed down now. She had a few things in her large purse, and hurriedly checked to see if her mother's money she sent was still there, It wasn't.

CHAPTER EIGHTEEN

Robin told Kym she could stay with Margaret, an AA friend of hers. But she also had some other good news: One of the places they perused together wanted Kym to help with office work, organize a newsletter for summer youth, and be the summer artistic director for minimum wage, It was better than nothing, and it was a start.

Kym praised God for not leaving her homeless, although she knew she could've probably gone home to Akron. Still, after the "Hooked" article, she really didn't want to go there just yet, and everybody she knew realized she had been sent to "the Big House". So she was very glad to at last have a chance in Ashtabula.

Margaret's house was clutter like none she'd ever seen before. There was no way anyone could even tell the color of the carpet because of clothes, papers, everything her granddaughter, age two, had heaped upon the place. Apparently the terrible twos were a reality, thought Kym. Just the same, Margaret and her daughter Jenny were very hospitable, and once a bed was found in the rooms upstairs, Kym had a place to temporarily stay,

She couldn't wait to start her new job, and looked forward to Monday with great earnestness. Finally the day came, and she was off and running or, better yet walking, because the bus was very close to Margaret's. She loved everything about the job, especially beginning a summer youth newsletter for a government agency that helps young people find jobs and learn skills of everyday life. She was contracted for three months and then she would have to find another job, because the contract was only for the summer. The newsletters, bulletin boards and filing she did were beyond reproach, and when the time came to leave, she nearly cried.

She had been hired as a church secretary, but after only three weeks was fired because she had been a felon. That's the way the ball and chain crumbles, she thought.

Then came a job she relished greatly, copyediting and proofreading the news in the Ashtabula Sun Times. What she didn't know is that she had attracted the attention of another reporter and copy editor named Alan. He finally made his presence known to her, and even though the last thing she wanted now was a boyfriend, she rather liked Alan. He was a bit overweight, but she was no shrinking violet, so that didn't really bother her,.

What she didn't know was that he had become the innocent victim of intimidation, the whipping boy, even though he did a great job, especially in reporting. But once she hooked up with him, the harassment began for her too, as often happens with the company one keeps, even if the company happens to be nice in most people's book.

The newspaper had no union, and reporters and other staff would call Alan and Kym names to their faces, behind their backs, and generally just made life miserable for them. When they became engaged, the hooting was even worse, Here were two decent people in an atmosphere of wolves. Once when Kym was asked to bring in a copy of her

'Hooked" article for the editor, Tom Freeborn, to read. He showed it to everyone after promising it would be kept strictly confidential. Kym as at lunch, and when she learned, the snickers and howls were too much for her to bear. It was now spring, and the article adorned Tom's office whenever she as out for some reason. Finally, Kym could stand the idiocy no longer. She put in her resignation after only six months. She thought she had found a job worthy of her talents but she was treated so shabbily that she could stand it no longer, and with a quiet "I quit," she was gone. Now where would she go for another job? Just rest on your laurels, girl, something will come along, I think. Alan stayed on to save for their upcoming marriage in July. Once before she left, she was accused of sending copy through on deadline and he was very nasty about it.

"Stop sending copy through, Kym!" She wasn't doing that, she was waiting for the machine to straighten up as it would do on its own, and she was trying to be a patient as she could. Then when the main troublemaker began to scream some more and approach her, she clenched her fists, and remembered the day she had decked that weasel from OPW. But after she cried, "Bob, don't you go postal on ME!" the jerk backed down. He never apologized, but he was a bit shaken and stirred after she gave him verbal hell. She was glad Alan could stand it better than she could, for there would only be his paycheck for a while to get them both through, Kym's mother had stopped sending her funds because she wanted her daughter to depend on Alan for support financially. She also had put two and two together and realized Kym was probably using some of those funds to buy cough syrup.

Alan stayed at the paper two or three more years, after they were married. They were wed on July 1, 1999, when Kym was 49 and Alan was 40. They never regretted such a serious move, and for the most part the marriage was a good one. Two things rocked it: Alan's firing, and Kym's continual addiction to Tussionex. Alan had suffered a problem with pornography, and had been warned by top brass at the paper not to use the company's Internet connection again while in the building. This was a problem he'd suffered even as a teenager, and he didn't listen to the warning. He called up some porn very quickly when he thought no one was around, but alas, one of the troublemakers was within eyeshot, and reported it to the editor, who took it to the publisher, and Alan was fired. No chance for explanations—just like Kym in her jail trial for those four years she did when she was clean. Life is so unfair, she thought.

He never called it up again, but it was never out of his system, he felt. Whether it was a direct attack on Kym's addiction, he never knew. But he abandoned it altogether after that fateful day.

Kym hoped her mom could come through with a little bit of money until she could find another job, and he could, too, she seemed to understand and sent them $500 to pay bills and for gas to look for new jobs. $500 to Kym was a real gift, because she knew once the Cable bill was paid they would have about $200 left over, and the gas bill wouldn't be due for another three weeks. She had plans for the money, and Alan knew it. But this time she didn't want to go get it herself, and go to a doctor. She wanted HIM to see someone. She pored through the physician sections of the phone book.

CHAPTER NINETEEN

"Honey, please do this for me. I'm out of my syrup and I'm starting withdrawal. When can you go?"

"Kym, do you know what you're asking? I'm freshly fired, and you want me to get something for you. What do you really think of me?"

"I think you're the best! But look, here are two internists who are open until 6 p.m. tonight. Could you try one? Please? I'm begging you, I really am."

"You told me about this damned addiction when we married, but I didn't know you'd have ME going to doctors for you. I can't, Kym. There's something very wrong about this."

"Yes, there is! My husband knows I'm heading into withdrawal and he refuses to help me! Thanks, stupid! Thanks for nothing!"

"Wha . . . aat? Are you serious? We aren't on medical coverage from the government yet and this is going to cost a lot of money, probably $90 for the visit, and $45 for the medicine, judging by what you've done so far. Can't you kick this? And I'm NOT stupid!"

"I swear, I'll divorce you if you don't go for me today. You owe me! You got fired and now the least you can do is to help me feel better! I won't take no for an answer."

"Then you will just have to leave me. I can't, Kym. Please, be reasonable. You are going back to that hellhole if you start this shit again. I know you've done it all along the time we've been married, but it has to stop NOW! And don't give me that sad-eyed little bunny look. Do something that's good for you for a change!"

"I hate you, I really do! You are so selfish, you blasted bastard! Why am I here instead of with someone else?"

"No one else would have you this way. It's the truth, Kym, I'm not trying to hurt you, but this is unacceptable."

"Fine, I'll go pack my things. I can stay with Robin the first night, Margaret then, and on my own after I get rid of you! Better get the papers from Atty. Fortier!"

"YOU get them! You're the one who's filing!"

"Please, Alan, just this once . . . I won't file. But please make me a little bit happier on this dismal day!"

"I've had enough! If weren't for your withdrawal, I might not want get more. But you win—just this ONCE. Okay? Once!"

"You're a doll, Alan! You're not stupid. Thanks soooo much! Look, here's an internist just a few blocks away. Could you . . . "

"Yes, yes, I'm a stupid dolt, right. But I can't stand that withdrawal and moaning around. So I'll go. Give me the name and address, and I'll get instant bronchitis."

"If you can't get syrup, change it to some kind of pain, because pills would be okay too, I found out the same stuff that's in Tussionex is in that Vicodin that's prescribed so much to people. So, just get pills or other syrup. Okay?"

'This is time out from my life, Kym. I hope you appreciate it."

You bet I do!" And she did.

This physician was a Dr. Castle, Richard Castle. Alan filled out all the papers and gave them to the receptionist,

"Oh, I'm so sorry you're sick, sir. But we'll help you as fast as possible."

'Thank you." Alan was really disturbed by Kym's addictive behavior. Hadn't jail taught her anything? Hadn't withdrawal taught her something> She must be nearly psychotic if she's wanting me to go to all these places. I don't want to get arrested either, he thought to himself, for very good reason. But everything came out as Kym had hoped it would. When He came from the pharmacy, he was carrying a five-ounce bottle of Tussionex. He entered the door and held it up to her.

"Oh, thanks, Babe! I knew you'd come through! You—uh—really DO have a mild sore throat, don't you?"

"C'mon. You don't have to pretend I'm really sick; that's just your dumb conscience. But here is your yellow shit, so have a ball!"

"I knew you'd do it! Don't worry—I won't keep this up. In a couple of weeks I'll be ready for rehab, and you can . . . "

"I don't want to hear it. You'll never be ready for rehab, not as long as you kept getting this crap, And as long as I am stupid enough to get it for you.;

"Oh, no, no! I really appreciate it, and I AM gonna quit soon. I can, I know I can."

"Yeah, and pigs can fly. Just amuse yourself, Kym. No one else wants to do it any more for you. Not me, not your mom, not the doctors, no one. Do you her me? NO ONE!"

Alan slammed the front door, turned to the bedroom and slammed that door too He couldn't do this much longer, if any longer. It was the same thing, time after time, and if the docs would refuse then Kym would really have massive withdrawal and more begging for him to go out again. No, he couldn't do this anymore. He may not be the syrup addicted individual, but he could be burned just the same if she ended up back in jail.

For the next four years, there was trip after trip to over 50 doctors and several counties once again. How Alan stood up no one will ever know, but Kym ended up once more back in the slammer, this time, luckily, for only six months. She just couldn't stop herself from taking pills, syrup, and asking for something called a fentanyl patch, which is a transdermal skin patch and a very strong opiate. Jail was similar to the time before, but only a much shorter scale, and she was grateful to get out. Still everything continued, she was hopelessly addicted and ready to kill herself because she was tired of lame braining it through euphoria, withdrawal, and the toll both were taking on her. If she didn't quit, she would land in prison yet another time. Finally, she ended up in a hospital rehab, and a miracle began that day.

CHAPTER TWENTY

Kym found herself at Hudson Hospital in Cleveland, Ohio, where she had come two days earlier. Detox took about five days, so she knew her time wasn't up yet. She felt weak, wanted her syrup, and hardly had an appetite. They were giving her valium to help her sleep, and they seemed to take the edge off withdrawal as well. But she knew that thus would just be another trip to the hospital, detox center, rehab center, or any other place she had to go when the going got rough.

She was given a shot of burdened, an opiate antagonist/agonist, or an opioid that helps keep the withdrawal at bay but does not produce euphoria in the process, She felt this was a better hospital than others she had detoxes inside But the best was yet to come.

A social worker named Becky had taken a special interest in her case, and wanted her to do as well as she possibly could, so after much deliberation and talks with other hospital officials, Kym was going to be given another chance on her fifty-seventh birthday, She was going to a methadone clinic. She had tried to get into one of two programs, suboxone and methadone, but the prior rehab hospital told her she was not suited for suboxone, They never told her why, and the physician who had studied her case came beaming into the room so excitedly that she was sure she was chosen. But his countenance fell, and he said she Wasn't the right type for it;;, whatever that meant.

As October 16 drew closer, she thought of one other birthday that was spent being transported to OPW, Now his was different. As her fifth day came up, she felt tired but not too bad inside, no withdrawal. It had all been finished by day five. What she would do is call a number the social worker gave her, come to the methadone clinic at 6 a.m., and be evaluated for eligibility into the program.

The gentleman who interviewed was a cheerful, older gentleman who loved to laugh, and when he took her information, he promised her she would be a client in the program. She was crying from happiness and joy. She had been an addict for over 22 years, and now there was hope. She was to come in the next day and learn about dosing, which was easy,

The Cleveland Treatment Center on Carnegie Avenue is where she chose to go, between the two downtown centers. She was glad she'd chosen it, because the personnel all seemed to be friendly and helpful, and above all – caring.

The next day she didn't have to be at the center until 9 a.m., She was taken to a window where she would be given an I.D. number and a small plastic cup of methadone. The usual dose is about thirty milligrams, then after physical and billing information is exchanged, the amount can be increased, Kym was on thirty milligrams at first, which was usually the starting dose, and she would go up eventually to about 110 mg., but not for several months.

Once the cup with the methadone was taken with fruit punch, it was filled again so that any remnant of methadone would not be lost in the glass, and the second glassful was taken, then the glass was thrown away, There would be no euphoria or strange behavior, but cravings and withdrawal would be very minimal from that day on.

Since that fateful day over two years ago, Kym has made many new friends at the clinic. She goes daily, which from Geneva is about 55 miles, but she receives gas vouches from the government, which makes the trip easier. She is editing a newsletter now about happenings at the clinic, whether awards are given to youth programs, parties are planned, clients and staff are recognized, and she does not deviate from that dose. There are no other opiates, no cough syrup or pain pills, or patches. Something has happened to Kym that hasn't happened to her ever before her 33rd birthday, She is happy, genuinely happy and content. She knows her dosage will eventually be tapered off, and from 110 mg. she is now at 60 and slowly coming down. Some patients have been on the program for many years, but Kym would rather not take that path, because someday soon she wants her whole life back, not just most of it. Alan is very happy at her progress also, and they do not have heated arguments any more.

There is one other thing that bears mentioning, and that is the lifeline Kym has received through this progressive program. The other thing about Kym and her story is that it is all true. She says a few minor details have been omitted, but all the important facts are here, I know this, because Kym's story is my story. I am Kym Corell in this book only. To all others I am Vonda Childress and I am glad.

www.ingramcontent.com/pod-product-compliance
Lightning Source LLC
Chambersburg PA
CBHW022133170526
45157CB00004B/1866